Oxford Case Histories in
Respiratory Medicine

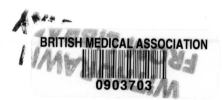

OXFORD CASE HISTORIES

Series Editors

Peter Rothwell and Sarah Pendlebury

Published:

Neurological Case Histories (Sarah Pendlebury and Peter Rothwell)
Oxford Case Histories in Gastroenterology and Hepatology (Alissa Walsh, Otto Buchel, Jane Collier, and Simon Travis)
Oxford Case Histories in Respiratory Medicine (John Stradling, Andrew Stanton, Najib Rahman, Annabel Nickol, and Helen Davies)

Forthcoming:

Oxford Case Histories in Cardiology (Colin Forfar, Javed Ehtisham and Rajkumar Rajendram)
Oxford Case Histories in Nephrology (Chris Pugh, Chris O'Callaghan, Aron Chakera, Richard Cornall and David Mole)
Oxford Case Histories in Rheumatology (Joel David, Anne Miller, Anushka Soni and Lyn Williamson)
Oxford Case Histories in Stroke and TIA (Sarah Pendlebury and Peter Rothwell)

Oxford Case Histories in Respiratory Medicine

John Stradling
Professor of Respiratory Medicine, Oxford University,
Consultant Physician, Oxford Centre for Respiratory
Medicine, Churchill Hospital, Oxford

Andrew Stanton
Specialist Registrar in Respiratory Medicine
Oxford Centre for Respiratory Medicine
Churchill Hospital, Oxford

Najib Rahman
Specialist Registrar and MRC Training Fellow
Oxford Centre for Respiratory Medicine
Churchill Hospital, Oxford

Annabel Nickol
Clinical Lecturer in Respiratory Medicine
Oxford Centre for Respiratory Medicine
Churchill Hospital, Oxford

Helen Davies
Specialist Registrar in Respiratory Medicine
Oxford Centre for Respiratory Medicine
Churchill Hospital, Oxford

OXFORD
UNIVERSITY PRESS

OXFORD
UNIVERSITY PRESS

Great Clarendon Street, Oxford OX2 6DP

Oxford University Press is a department of the University of Oxford.
It furthers the University's objective of excellence in research, scholarship,
and education by publishing worldwide in

Oxford New York

Auckland Cape Town Dar es Salaam Hong Kong Karachi
Kuala Lumpur Madrid Melbourne Mexico City Nairobi
New Delhi Shanghai Taipei Toronto

With offices in

Argentina Austria Brazil Chile Czech Republic France Greece
Guatemala Hungary Italy Japan Poland Portugal Singapore
South Korea Switzerland Thailand Turkey Ukraine Vietnam

Oxford is a registered trade mark of Oxford University Press
in the UK and in certain other countries

Published in the United States
by Oxford University Press Inc., New York
© Oxford University Press, 2010

The moral rights of the author have been asserted
Database right Oxford University Press (maker)

First published 2010

British Library Cataloguing in Publication Data

Data available

Library of Congress Cataloging in Publication Data

Data available

Typeset in Minion by Cepha Imaging Private Ltd., Bangalore, India
Printed in Great Britain
on acid-free paper by
CPI Antony Rowe

ISBN 978-0-19-955637-3 (Pbk.)

10 9 8 7 6 5 4 3 2 1

A note from the series editors

Case histories have always had an important role in medical education, but most published material has been directed at undergraduates or residents. The Oxford Case Histories series aims to provide more complex case-based learning for clinicians in specialist training and consultants, with a view to aiding preparation for entry and exit-level specialty examinations or revalidation. Each case book follows the same format with approximately 50 cases, each comprising a brief clinical history and investigations, followed by questions on differential diagnosis and management, and detailed answers with discussion. All cases are peer-reviewed by Oxford consultants in the relevant specialty. At the end of each book, cases are listed by mode of presentation, aetiology and diagnosis.

We are grateful to our colleagues in the various medical specialties for their enthusiasm and hard work in making the series possible.

Sarah Pendlebury and Peter Rothwell

Quotes on the first book in the series – "Neurological Case Histories"

"I recommend this excellent volume highly .... this book will enlighten and entertain consultants, and all readers will learn something."

Lancet Neurology 2007; 6: 951

"This short and well-written text is .... designed to enhance the reader's diagnostic ability and clinical understanding .... A well documented and practical book"

European Journal of Neurology 2007; 14: e19

Introduction

Postgraduate medical education has changed considerably over the last 30 years. There is greater emphasis on structured learning, but apprenticeship time has decreased. Thus specialist registrars may reach the end of their training without having seen cases of either rare diseases, rare presentations of common diseases or unusual problems in association with common diseases. Most physicians learn from cases they have seen. This collection of cases is a second-best alternative, providing vignettes that hopefully will come to mind when a similar case is encountered in the future.

The cases are not meant to comprehensively cover the 'syllabus' of a specialist registrar in respiratory medicine, but are selected for their interest, or to elucidate points that the authors feel are important but may be under-appreciated. The style of presentation thus inevitably varies depending on the type of message and some of the problems discussed have no right answer, ours may well be disputed!

We hope the question-and-answer format will keep the reader on their toes and make reading through the cases more fun.

Acknowledgements

Many people have given their time to read through these cases and correct errors or improve clarity. We are very grateful for their input; in particular Rachel Benamore has provided considerable help with the radiology, and Rolf Smith read through all the cases to provide us with invaluable help. These are the individuals who reviewed one or more cases for us: Lesley Bennett, Malcolm Benson, Di Bilton, Steve Chapman, Sonya Craig, Ling-Pei Ho, Rob Davies, Colin Forfar, Maxine Hardinge, Robin Howard, Gary Lee, Raashid Luqmani, Lorna McWilliam, Grace Robinson, Rana Sayeed, Claire Shovlin, Catherine Swales, Catherine Thomas, Chris Winearls, and John Wrightson. Needless to say any errors remain our responsibility.

Contents

Abbreviations

AAFB	Acid- and alcohol-fast bacilli	CTEPH	Chronic thromboembolic pulmonary hypertension
ABG	Arterial blood gases	CTPA	Computerized tomographic pulmonary angiogram
ABPA	Allergic bronchopulmonary aspergillosis	CVID	Common variable immunodeficiency
ACE	Angiotensin converting enzyme	CXR	Chest radiograph
ANA	Anti-nuclear antibody	DBP	Diastolic blood pressure
ANCA	Anti-nuclear cytoplasmic antibody	DCT	Direct Coombs test
ARDS	Adult respiratory distress syndrome	DNA	Deoxyribonucleic acid
		DOT	Directly observed therapy
ASD	Atrial septal defect	DPB	Diffuse panbronchiolitis
AVM	Arteriovenous malformation	DVLA	Driver vehicle licensing authority
BAL	Bronchoalveolar lavage		
BAPE	Benign asbestos-related pleural effusion	DVT	Deep vein thrombosis
		EIA	Enzyme immunoassay
BE	Base excess	ELCs	Emphysema-like changes
BMI	Body mass index (kgs/metre^2)	ELS	extralobar sequestration
BMT	Bone marrow transplant	EPP	extrapleural pneumonectomy
BNP	Brain natriuretic peptide	ESS	Epworth sleepiness score
BO	bronchiolitis obliterans	FEV$_1$	Forced expiratory volume in one second
BPM	Beats per minute		
Ca^{++}	Calcium	FRC	Functional residual volume
CBG	Capillary blood gases	FVC	Forced expiratory volume
CCAM	Congenital cystic adenomatoid malformation	GVHD	Graft-versus-host-disease
		H&E	Haematoxylin and Eosin
CETTE	Contrast-enhanced transthoracic echo	Hb	Haemoglobin
		[HCO$_3$]$^-$	Bicarbonate
CF	Cystic fibrosis	HES	Hypereosinophilic syndrome
CFTR	Cystic fibrosis transmembrane conductance regulator	HGV	Heavy goods vehicle
		HHT	Hereditary haemorrhagic telangiectasia
CLL	Chronic lymphatic leukaemia		
COP	Cryptogenic organizing pneumonia	HIV	Human immunodeficiency virus
		HLA	Human leukocyte antigen
CPAP	Continuous positive airway pressure	HP	Hypersensitivity pneumonitis
		HPS	Hepatopulmonary syndrome
CRP	C-reactive protein		
CT	Computerized tomography		

HRCT	High resolution computerized tomography	OSA	Obstructive sleep apnoea
HR	Heart rate	OSAS	Obstructive sleep apnoea syndrome
ICS	Inhaled corticosteroid	OSLER	Oxford sleep resistance test
IL1	Interleukin 1	PA	Pulmonary artery
ILS	intralobar sequestration	P_aCO_2	Partial pressure of arterial carbon-dioxide
INR	International normalized ratio		
IPF	Interstitial pulmonary fibrosis	P_aO_2	Partial pressure of arterial oxygen
IVC	Inferior vena cava		
JVP	Jugular venous pressure	PAP	Pulmonary artery pressure
K^+	Potassium	PAVM	Pulmonary arteriovenous malformations
K_{CO}	Carbon-monoxide transfer coefficient	PCD	Primary ciliary dyskinesia
LAM	Lymphangioleiomyomatosis	PCR	Protein creatinine ratio
LCH	Langerhans cell histiocytosis	PEFR	Peak expiratory flow rate
LDH	Lactate dehydrogenase	PH	Pulmonary hypertension
LFTs	Liver function tests	PFO	Patent foramen ovale
LIP	Lymphoid interstitial pneumonia	PFTs	Pulmonary function tests
		PND	Post-nasal drip or paroxysmal nocturnal dyspnoea
LTOT	Long-term oxygen therapy		
LV	Left ventricle	PSP	Primary spontaneous pneumothorax
LVSF	Left ventricular systolic function		
		RA-ILD	Rheumatoid associated interstitial lung disease
MAC	Mycobacteria avium complex		
MCS	Microscopy, culture and sensitivity	RAW	Airway resistance (from body box)
MCT	Medium-chain triglycerides	RBILD	Respiratory bronchiolitis–interstitial lung disease
MCV	Mean corpuscular volume		
MDR-TB	Multi-drug resistant TB	RPO	Re-expansion pulmonary oedema
MGUS	Monoclonal gammopathy of unknown significance		
		RV	Residual volume/Right ventricle
MI	Myocardial infarction		
MPO	Myeloperoxidase	S_aO_2	Arterial oxygen saturations
MSLT	Multiple sleep latency test	SBP	Systolic blood pressure
MWT	Maintenance of wakefulness test	SOB	Shortness of breath
		SVC	Superior vena cava
Na^+	Sodium	T4	Thyroxine
NSAID	Non-steroidal anti-inflammatory agent	TB	Tuberculosis
		TBB	Transbronchial biopsy
NICE	National Institute for Health and Clinical Excellence	TLC	Total lung capacity
		TL_{CO}	Carbon-monoxide transfer factor
NSIP	Non-specific interstitial pneumonia		
		TNM	Tumour/nodes/metastases classification
NTM	Non-tuberculous mycobacteria		

TPN	Total parenteral nutrition	USS	Ultrasound scan
U&Es	Urea and electrolytes	VATS	Video-assisted thoracoscopy
UACS	Upper airway cough syndrome	VCD	Vocal cord dysfunction
		VTE	Venous thrombo-embolism
UIP	Usual interstitial pneumonia	V/Q	Ventilation/perfusion

Normal ranges

	Lower limit	Upper limit	units
Hb (men)	13	18	g/dL
Hb (women)	11.5	15	g/dL
MCV	83	105	fL
WCC	4	11	$\times 10^9$/L
Neutrophils	2	7	$\times 10^9$/L
Lymphocytes	1	4	$\times 10^9$/L
Eosinophils	0.02	0.5	$\times 10^9$/L
Platelets	150	400	$\times 10^9$/L
PTT	10	14	s
APTT	22	34	s
ESR	0	about half the age	mm/hr
Na	135	145	mmol/L
K	3.5	5	mmol/L
Urea	2.5	6.7	mmol/L
Creatinine	70	150	umol/L
Bilirubin	3	17	umol/L
AST	3	35	IU/L
ALT	10	45	IU/L
ALP	75	250	IU/L
Albumin	35	50	g/L
GGT (men)	11	51	IU/L
GGT (women)	7	33	IU/L
Ca (corr)	2.12	2.62	mmol/L
PO_4	0.8	1.45	mmol/L
Glucose (fasting)	3.5	5.5	mmol/L
CRP	0	8	mg/L
ACE	18	55	IU/L
α1 anti trypsin	107	209	mg/dL
PSA	0	4	ng/mL
PaO_2	12	14	kPa
$PaCO_2$	4.7	5.9	kPa
pH	7.36	7.44	
Base excess	−2	2	meq/L
Bicarbonate	23	27	meq/L
IgG	6	13	g/L
IgA	0.8	3	g/L
IgM	0.4	2.5	g/L
IgE	5	120	kU/L

Case 1

A 42-year-old lady was referred for respiratory review with a history of asthma, which had become difficult to control over the last 3 years, with increased nocturnal cough and peak flow variability. She had received multiple courses of oral antibiotics and steroids to which she would briefly respond, and was on a long-term combined inhaled steroid and long-acting beta agonist. She used a nasal steroid for nasal polyps. She had not moved house or changed jobs, she worked as a gardener and had no pets.

Questions

1a) What reasons could explain this deterioration after many years of good control?

Answers

1a) What reasons could explain this deterioration after many years of good control?

There are multiple reasons to fail to respond to asthma therapy, including a poor inhaler technique or adherence to therapy. Reasons for deterioration in symptoms after good control include:

- Development of oesophageal reflux
- New exposure to asthma triggers, e.g. house-dust-mite, cat fur, pollen or occupational exposure
- New psychological or social pressure
- Alternative diagnoses, such as the development of allergic bronchopulmonary aspergillosis (ABPA) or Churg–Strauss syndrome
- Gain in weight.

Investigations showed

- Full blood count: Hb, 13.5g/dL
- WCC, 7.29×10^9/L
- Eosinophils, 3.21×10^9/L
- Platelets, 362×10^9/L
- Total IgE, 620 ng/ml (normal range 5–120)
- *Aspergillus* RAST (IgE), strongly positive
- *Aspergillus* precipitins (IgG), 2 lines (where 1 line = weakly positive and 6 = strongly positive)
- Sputum culture, mucoid *Pseudomonas aeruginosa*
- CF genetic screening, negative for common CF mutations.

Questions

1b) What do the CXR and CT scan in Fig. 1.1 show?

1c) What diagnosis do investigations support?

1d) What are the typical clinical features of this condition?

1e) Discuss treatments options for this lady.

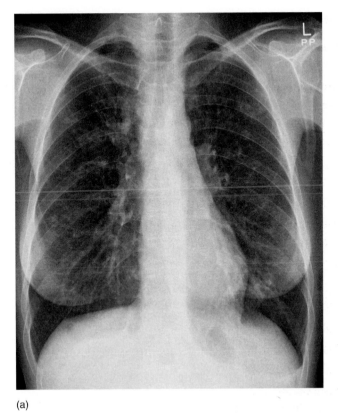

(a)

(b)

Fig. 1.1 (a) CXR and (b) CT chest.

Answers

1b) What do the CXR and CT scan in Fig. 1.1 show?

The CXR shows hyper-expanded lung fields, with widespread bronchiectatic changes. The CT slice shows dilated airways, much larger than the adjacent blood vessel, in keeping with bronchiectasis. There is also 'tree in bud nodularity', which may be suggestive of small airway chronic or atypical infection.

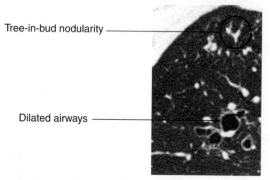

Tree-in-bud nodularity

Dilated airways

Fig. 1.2 Portion of CT-chest illustrating features in keeping with allergic bronchopulmonary aspergillosis.

1c) What diagnosis do investigations support?

Investigations support a diagnosis of allergic bronchopulmonary aspergillosis, ABPA. Atopic patients with asthma and cystic fibrosis with IgE-mediated allergy to inhaled *Aspergillus* spores are vulnerable to this condition. They may develop IgE and IgG reactions to *Aspergillus* in the airways, provoking mucous plugging with distal consolidation, and then ABPA, with inflammatory damage to the airways and resultant bronchiectasis. Damp conditions, composting organic material and thunderstorms are associated with high *Aspergillus* spore counts, and so may lead to exacerbations. Since simple atopic asthma is at one end of a continuum, with ABPA at the other, there is no single diagnostic test that defines the transition. The presence of the features in Box 1.1 would support the diagnosis, with the first four being the most important. Many asthmatics and patients with cystic fibrosis have one or more findings suggestive of ABPA, but do not fulfil all criteria listed.

ABPA is a complex hypersensitivity reaction, often in patients with asthma or cystic fibrosis that occurs when bronchi become colonized by *Aspergillus*.

Box 1.1 Diagnostic features of ABPA

- Longstanding history of asthma
- Immediate positive IgE reaction to *Aspergillus* on skin testing, or on serum testing using RAST (radioallergosorbent test)
- Precipitating serum IgG antibodies to *Aspergillus fumigatus*
- Central bronchiectasis on chest CT
- Peripheral blood eosinophilia
- Serum total IgE concentration elevated > 1000ng/mL
- Flitting lung infiltrates on CXR or chest HRCT.

Repeated episodes of bronchial obstruction, inflammation, and mucoid impaction can lead to bronchiectasis, fibrosis and respiratory compromise. It is thought healthy, unaffected individuals are able to effectively eliminate fungal spores. They have low levels of IgG against fungal antigens in the circulation, and low anti-fungal secretory IgA in bronchoalveolar fluid. In contrast, exposure of atopic individuals to fungal spores or mycelial fragments results in the formation of IgE and IgG antibodies. *Aspergillus* responsive T-cells generate the cytokines interleukin (IL)-4, IL-5 and IL-13, which account for the eosinophilia and raised IgE in ABPA. *Aspergillus* colonization of the asthmatic airway leads to vigorous IgE- and IgG-mediated immune responses superimposed on the asthmatic milieu. In spite of these vigorous responses in ABPA, the fungus is able to colonize the airway and cause recurrent symptoms. Proteolytic enzymes are released by *Aspergillus* as part of its exophytic feeding strategy, and these enzymes may in theory damage airway walls. However, exuberant host defence mechanisms are thought to be the dominant method of damage, hence there is a good response to steroids. Spores and hyphae (indicating germination of the spores in the airway) are sometimes seen on direct microscopy, and *Aspergillus* is cultured from sputum in up to two-thirds of patients with ABPA. As in most cases of ABPA, the patient in this case had a background history of atopic asthma.

1d) **What are the typical clinical features of this condition?**

Typical clinical features of ABPA are long-standing asthma with a more recent deterioration, complicated by recurrent episodes of bronchial obstruction and expectoration of brownish mucous plugs, fever, malaise, peripheral blood eosinophilia and sometimes episodic haemoptysis.

Wheezing is not always present, and some patients present with asymptomatic 'flitting' pulmonary consolidation.

1e) **Discuss treatment options for this lady.**

Treatment of ABPA involves optimal care of bronchiectasis and asthma, plus early use of oral steroids and consideration of itraconazole with drug level monitoring where this is available. This needs to be prescribed for 3 to 6 months (regular liver function tests are needed as the drug may be hepatotoxic) and the IgG levels to *Aspergillus* should fall with fungal load reduction. Inhaled steroids may help control symptoms of asthma, but do not have documented efficacy in preventing acute episodes of ABPA.

Further reading

Denning D, O'Driscoll B, Hogaboam C, Bowyer P and Niven RM (2006). The link between fungi and severe asthma: a summary of the evidence. *Eur Respir J*; **27**: 615–626.

Stevens DA, Schwartz HJ, Lee JY, Moskovitz BL, Jerome DC, Catanzaro A *et al.* (2000). A randomized trial of itraconazole in allergic bronchopulmonary aspergillosis. *New Eng J Med*; **342**: 756–762.

Case 2

A 77-year-old lady was referred with progressive breathlessness over 3 years. She was breathless walking 100 yards on the flat and could not manage stairs. There were no other respiratory symptoms. Past history was of myocardial infarction (MI) in 1984, and duodenal ulcer 1988. She had stopped smoking after her MI, with a prior 40 pack year smoking history. Her medication consisted of simvastatin, lisinopril, furosemide, aspirin, amiodarone, salbutamol and omeprazole. All of her cardiac medications were commenced post-MI. She kept no pets. On examination there was central cyanosis, finger clubbing and resting oxygen saturations of 83% on room air. JVP was not elevated and there was no peripheral oedema. Cardiac examination revealed an aortic sclerotic murmur and respiratory examination revealed bibasal fine inspiratory crackles in the lower zones. Abdominal and musculoskeletal examination was unremarkable.

Investigations

- Hb 14.3g/dL, WCC 5.94 × 10^9/L (eosinophils 0.18 × 10^9/L), platelets 145 × 10^9/L
- ESR, 48mm/h
- U&Es, normal
- Bilirubin 39 µmol/L, ALT 18 IU/L, ALP 308 IU/L
- Albumin, 27g/L
- Rheumatoid factor, 69.4U (<10, negative; 10–30, borderline; >30, positive)
- ANA, anti-smooth muscle antibody, anti-mitochondrial antibody, and anti-gastric parietal cell antibody: negative
- Alpha 1 antitrypsin, 185mg/dL (normal 107–209 mg/dL)
- ABG (on air), PaO_2 6.7 kPa, $PaCO_2$ 4.17 kPa, $[HCO_3]^-$ 23.3 mol/L, pH 7.45
- ECG, normal
- Abdominal USS, liver appeared slightly enlarged with an irregular outline. Spleen was also slightly irregular. Pancreas and kidneys were normal.

Table 2.1 Pulmonary function tests

	Measured	% Predicted
$FEV_1(L)$	2.0	131
FVC(L)	2.8	144
$FEV_1/FVC(\%)$	71	
FRC(L)	2.8	110
RV(L)	1.9	97
TLC(L)	4.7	108
VA(L)	3.6	82
TL_{CO}(mmol/min/kPa)	2.05	34
K_{CO}(mmol/min/kPa/L)	0.57	41

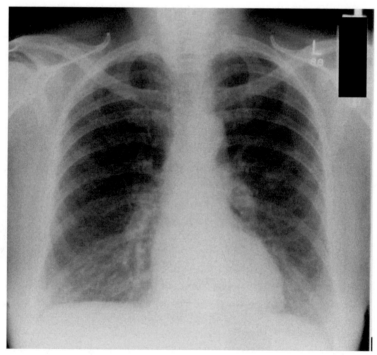

Fig. 2.1 CXR.

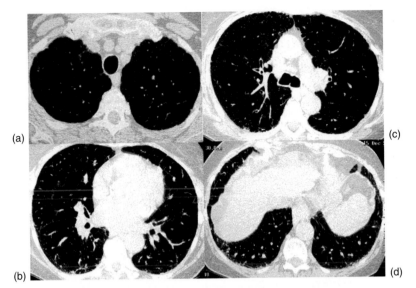

(a)

(b)

(c)

(d)

Fig. 2.2 HRCT thorax.

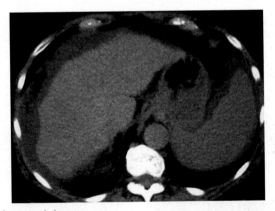

Fig. 2.3 CT of upper abdomen.

Questions

2a) Interpret the lung function tests.

2b) Interpret the CXR.

2c) Interpret the CT images.

2d) What specific diagnoses can be made from the above investigations?

2e) What further diagnoses should be considered, what simple bedside test can help with the differential, and what further investigations are needed?

Answers

2a) **Interpret the lung function tests.**

The pulmonary function tests (PFT's) show slightly supra-normal dynamic lung volumes (although in more elderly patients prediction of 'normal' is less well defined), but no evidence of any obstructive or restrictive ventilatory defect. In addition the static lung volumes are also normal. There is an isolated marked reduction in gas transfer but the cause cannot be deduced.

2b) **Interpret the CXR.**

The CXR (Fig. 2.1) shows bilateral basal reticulonodular opacities. Otherwise there is no focal lung lesion, the heart size and mediastinal contours are normal. The right hemi-diaphragm is slightly flat in appearance.

2c) **Interpret the CT images.**

The HRCT (Fig. 2.2) shows moderate emphysematous changes most marked in the mid and upper zones (Fig. 2.4b). There are minor degrees of subpleural reticulation and honeycombing at both bases (Fig. 2.4a). On the abdominal image (Fig. 2.3) the liver has an irregular margin and there is splenomegaly. There is also ascites present.

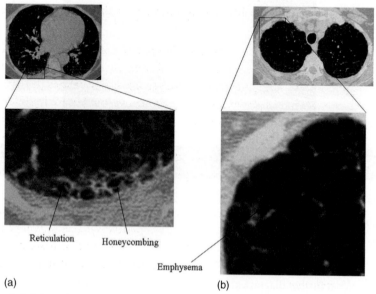

Reticulation   Honeycombing

Emphysema

(a)   (b)

Fig. 2.4 Enlarged portions of HRCT.

2d) **What specific diagnoses can be made from the above investigations?**

CT diagnoses (Fig. 2.4) are:

- Emphysema
- Interstitial lung disease (likely idiopathic pulmonary fibrosis, UIP pattern on CT)
- Cirrhosis with portal hypertension.

At this point the investigations are not compatible with a unifying respiratory diagnosis. The degree of emphysema and interstitial lung disease identified on the CT seems out of proportion to the hypoxaemia on the blood gases. Furthermore, the lung function shows no evidence of obstructive or restrictive defects. The isolated reduction in gas transfer could be due to emphysema or early interstitial lung disease, but again this is marked (41% predicted) and one would perhaps expect greater physiological disturbance were either, or both, of these two diagnoses primarily responsible. The finger clubbing could be caused by the interstitial lung disease or possibly cirrhosis. The presence of honeycombing suggests established fibrosis, the precise cause of which cannot be absolutely certain. Amiodarone could potentially be implicated and it would not be unreasonable for this to be stopped, but again it is certainly unlikely to be the whole story.

2e) **What further diagnoses should be considered, what simple bedside test can help with the differential, and what further investigations are needed?**

A full explanation for her respiratory failure and markedly low gas transfer is needed. Given the presence of cirrhosis with ascites, the hepatopulmonary syndrome with pulmonary arteriovenous malformations (AVMs) is the most likely unifying diagnosis. An alternative, but less likely explanation, would be chronic pulmonary thromboembolic disease. A simple bedside test to help sort this out would be to investigate any postural changes in oxygen saturations. In pulmonary AVMs, oxygen saturation may fall on assuming an upright posture (orthodeoxia). Confirmatory investigations would therefore be:

(i) Whole chest CT pulmonary angiogram. This showed no evidence of pulmonary emboli. Increased nodularity was seen peripherally at both bases (arrows, Fig. 2.5), which would be consistent with arteriovenous malformations secondary to hepatopulmonary syndrome.

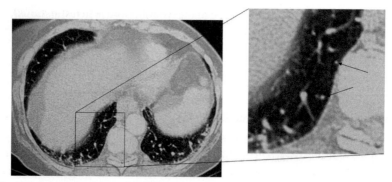

Fig. 2.5 Enlarged portion of CTPA.

   (ii) 'Shuntogram' using [99m]technicium-microaggregated albumin lung perfusion scanning. This demonstrated renal uptake of 17% of radiolabelled microalbumin administered, consistent with a shunt (see Case 40).

Hepatopulmonary syndrome (HPS)

This is defined by the triad of liver disease (most commonly cirrhosis, although cases with acute and chronic non-cirrhotic hepatitis have been described), intrapulmonary vasodilation at capillary and pre-capillary level (producing right to left shunting) and impaired arterial oxygenation. Pathogenesis is unclear but is thought to relate to increased pulmonary production of nitric oxide in liver disease. HPS should be considered in any patient with liver disease who has unexplained breathlessness and arterial deoxygenation. The phenomenon of orthodeoxia, a significant decrease of PaO_2 or SaO_2 going from supine to upright position, is explained by postural redirection of pulmonary blood flow to mainly the bases where the AVMs predominate; this increases the effective shunting compared to a horizontal posture, where pulmonary blood flow is more evenly distributed. Because these dilated vessels are still adjacent to alveoli, and not anatomically separate vascular malformations, they do not behave quite as true shunts. However, hypoxia develops through a mechanism called 'diffusion–perfusion impairment', whereby oxygen molecules cannot diffuse in time to the centre of dilated capillaries from adjacent alveoli to oxygenate haemoglobin in erythrocytes at the centre of the stream of blood. It is thought this is also aggravated by a hyperdynamic circulation, resulting in a shorter transit time through the lungs for the red cell. This also explains why increasing inspired oxygen concentration raises the PaO_2 more than would be expected with a true shunt.

Diagnosis of HPS is best made by either contrast-enhanced transthoracic echo (CETTE) or ^{99m}technicium-microaggregated albumin perfusion scanning. With CETTE, microbubbles (injected peripherally) appearing abnormally in the *left* atrium, after at least three cardiac cycles, implies an intrapulmonary shunt (immediate appearance in the left heart implies intra-cardiac right-to-left shunt). With isotope perfusion scanning, the pulmonary vasculature should trap the majority (94–97%) of the 20–60μm-diameter albumin microaggregates, with extrapulmonary uptake only appearing in brain, liver or kidney if there is right-to-left shunting. In HPS, the shunt ratio is over 10% and can be as high as 70%, but this will not differentiate between intrapulmonary or intra-cardiac shunting, of course.

Patients with HPS and cirrhosis have markedly reduced survival compared to those without (median survival 10.6 versus 40.8 months), and HPS is recognized as an added indication for liver transplant in some centres. Some case reports demonstrate complete resolution of HPS following transplant, but no other treatment is of proven benefit. There are isolated case reports of benefit from coil embolization and transjugular intraheptic portosystemic shunting. Supplementary oxygen can improve oxygenation and symptoms.

Further reading

Shenk P (2005). The hepatopulmonary syndrome. *ERJ Monograph* **34**, chapter 7.

Case 3

A 41-year-old woman presented with a 4-month history of shortness of breath on exertion, with no associated cough or systemic symptoms. Her previous medical history included Raynaud's phenomenon, and 18 months dysphagia and dyspepsia. A recent barium swallow demonstrated severe oesophageal dysmotility and inco-ordination of the gastro-oesophageal junction. She smoked (20-pack year smoking history), and was overweight (body mass index 43). Examination was normal, apart from skin changes of hands and mouth (Fig. 3.1). Pulmonary function tests (Table 3.1), a CT chest (Fig. 3.2) and an echocardiogram were performed. She had a modestly elevated pulmonary arterial pressure at 35mmHg.

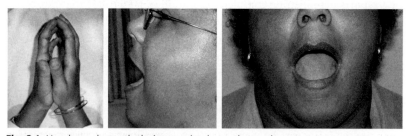

Fig. 3.1 Hands, and mouth during maximal mouth opening.

Table 3.1 Pulmonary function tests

	Measured	% Predicted
SaO$_2$	94–96%	
FEV$_1$(L)	1.9L	71
FVC(L)	2.4L	75
FEV$_1$/FVC ratio	82%	
FRC(L)	2.2L	79
RV(L)	1.6L	92
TLC(L)	3.9L	83
TL$_{CO}$(mmol/min/kPa)	4.51	50
K$_{CO}$(mmol/min/kPa/L)	1.43	76

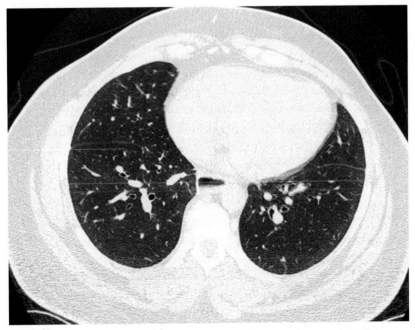

Fig. 3.2 CT chest.

Questions

3a) Describe the changes shown in Figs 3.1 and 3.2.

3b) Describe the abnormalities shown by the pulmonary function tests. List two causes of the restrictive defect observed in this patient and suggest how you could tell which one predominates.

3c) Suggest a unifying diagnosis.

Answers

3a) **Describe the changes shown in Figs 3.1 and 3.2.**

Skin changes: Fig. 3.1 shows changes consistent with scleroderma, with skin tightening, induration and thickening around finger tips and mouth. HRCT changes; Fig. 3.2 shows subtle sub-pleural ground glass opacification, without significant associated reticulation or traction bronchial dilation.

3b) **Describe the abnormalities shown by the pulmonary function tests. List two causes of the restrictive defect observed in this patient and suggest how you could tell which one predominates.**

Pulmonary function tests (Table 3.1). Restrictive spirometry is demonstrated, with a raised FEV_1/FVC ratio, proportional reduction of static lung volumes, and low KCO. Two potential causes of this patient's restrictive spirometry are interstitial lung disease and obesity. If obesity were the primary cause and the underlying lungs were normal, then KCO would be supra-normal (Hart *et al.* 2002). However, in this case the KCO is significantly reduced at 76% predicted, which implies the underlying lung parenchyma is abnormal and interstitial lung disease predominates.

3c) **Suggest a unifying diagnosis.**

Systemic sclerosis. Scleroderma, Raynaud's phenomenon, oesophageal dysmotility and possible early interstitial lung disease are suggestive of diffuse cutaneous systemic sclerosis. Systemic sclerosis is a generalized connective tissue disorder occurring more commonly in women.

Question

3d) There are two subsets of systemic sclerosis: limited cutaneous systemic sclerosis and diffuse cutaneous systemic sclerosis. What features distinguish them?

Answer

3d) **There are two subsets of systemic sclerosis: limited cutaneous systemic sclerosis and diffuse cutaneous systemic sclerosis. What features distinguish them?**
See Table 3.2.

Table 3.2 Comparison of the two sub-types of systemic sclerosis

Feature	Form of cutaneous systemic sclerosis	
	Limited (formerly called CREST syndrome)	**Diffuse**
Raynaud's phenomenon	Present for years, and may be severe	Occurs within one year of skin changes
Skin changes	Limited to hands, face, feet and forearms or absent. Late skin calcification and telangiectasia may occur	Widespread skin involvement of both trunk and extremities
Nails	Dilated nail fold capillary loops	Nail fold capillary dilatation and capillary destruction
Pulmonary changes	A significant late incidence of pulmonary hypertension with or without interstitial lung disease	Early and significant incidence of interstitial lung disease
Other organ damage	A significant late incidence of trigeminal neuralgia and liver disease	Early and significant incidence of oliguric renal failure, diffuse gastrointestinal disease and myocardial infarction
Antibodies	A high incidence of anti-centromere antibody (70–80% of patients)	Anti-Scl-70 (antitopoisomerase I) antibody positive (30% of patients). Presence associated with interstitial lung disease, and general disease activity

Questions

3e) How should patients be monitored?

3f) Suggest treatment options.

Answers

3e) **How should patients be monitored?**

Patients with systemic sclerosis affecting the heart, lungs or kidneys require specialist and multi-disciplinary follow-up, and may need regular pulmonary function testing, echocardiography for estimation of pulmonary arterial pressures and renal function tests. Identification of patients at risk is difficult, as the disease may be quiescent for long periods.

The decision to start treatment is often difficult, as many patients have limited disease that may not progress. Factors prompting initiation of treatment are:

- Deterioration in serial pulmonary function tests or CXR over the last 6–12 months
- Severe respiratory disease (extensive disease on CT, moderate to severe reduction in TL_{CO} or restrictive ventilatory defect)
- Duration of systemic disease <5 years (especially <2 years)
- Anti-Scl-70 (antitopoisomerase I) antibody positivity
- Prominent ground glass attenuation on HRCT without traction bronchial dilation or reticulation.

3f) **Suggest treatment options.**

Most randomized clinical trials have been small ($n<40$), and, due to the heterogenous nature of systemic sclerosis, results are difficult to generalize. In view of this, treatment of patients with severe disease is often based on expert opinion rather than randomized, controlled trial data. Due to the equivocal clinical benefit, side-effects, cost, inconvenient routes of delivery of some drugs, therapy is often not given to those with mild disease.

In interstitial lung disease, intra-venous or oral cyclophosphamide, and low-dose prednisolone are treatments of first choice. These tend to be continued for one year, before converting to prednisolone and azathioprine.

In pulmonary hypertension, a combination of calcium antagonists, sildenafil and an endothelin receptor antagonist (e.g. bosentan) are often used in combination. Referral of patients with pulmonary hypertension to a specialist centre should be made.

Calcium channel blockers, such as nifedipine, may be used to treat symptoms of Raynaud's phenomenon, although they do not reverse skin changes, and may worsen oesophageal dysmotility. An alternative option is topical glycerol trinitrate paste.

The prostacyclin analogues, e.g. inhaled iloprost, oral beraprost and subcutaneous treprostinil, have been shown to have a beneficial effect on the vascular manifestations of systemic sclerosis, including both pulmonary hypertension (associated with significant improvements in various pulmonary function, 6-minute walk test and dyspnoea index) and Raynaud's phenomenon. Monthly dexamethasone injections may also have a modest beneficial effect on pulmonary function tests and frequency of Raynaud's attacks. Low-dose oral prednisolone is sometimes used, although high doses tend to be avoided due to the possible risk of renal crisis, a rare complication of scleroderma, through an unknown mechanism. Other agents, such as methotrexate, azathioprine, interferons and antioxidants, have not been shown to have a significant beneficial effect.

Further reading
Scleroderma lung disease

Henness S and Wigley F (2007). Current drug therapy for scleroderma and secondary Raynaud's phenomenon: evidence-based review. *Curr Opinion Rheum*; **19**: 611–618.

Highland K and Silver R (2005). New developments in scleroderma interstitial lung disease. *Curr Opin Rheumatol*; **17**: 737–745.

Latsi P and Wells A (2003). Evaluation and management of alveolitis and interstitial lung disease. *Curr Opin Rheumatol*; **15**: 748–755.

Tashkin D, Elashoff R, Clements P *et al.* (2006). Cyclophosphamide versus placebo in scleroderma lung disease. *N Engl J Med*; **345**: 2655–2666.

Supra-normal carbon monoxide transfer factor in restrictive lung disease

Hart N, Cramer D, Ward S *et al.* (2002). Effect of pattern and severity of respiratory muscle weakness on carbon monoxide gas transfer and lung volumes. *Eur Respir J*; **20**: 1–7.

Case 4

A 42-year-old Caucasian female was referred with a cough. She had been diagnosed with asthma 6 years previously on the basis of a recurrent cough, productive of clear or purulent sputum, and exertional breathlessness; she had no history of wheeze and her peak flow values did not vary significantly.

She had been treated with high-dose inhaled corticosteroids and long acting beta-2 agonists with little benefit, and a course of oral prednisolone was unhelpful. A 3-month trial of proton pump inhibitor therapy also gave no relief. She did intermittently use topical nasal steroids for sinusitis but had noticed no impact on her cough. She had never smoked.

On examination her SaO_2 was 98% on air. She had crackles in both mid-zones on auscultation but no wheeze. Her pulmonary function tests are shown in Table 4.1 (NB Patient coughed during expiratory manoeuvres).

Table 4.1 Pulmonary function tests

	Measured	% Predicted
PEFR(L/min)	270	85
$FEV_1(L)$	1.4	71
FVC (L)	2.3	75
FEV_1/FVC ratio (%)	59	
VA(L)	3.6	78
TL_{CO}(mmol/min/kPa)	3.58	55
K_{CO}(mmol/min/kPa/L)	1.01	71
No change following administration of 5mg nebulized salbutamol		

Her CXR was normal and a thoracic CT was arranged (basal slices, Fig. 4.1).

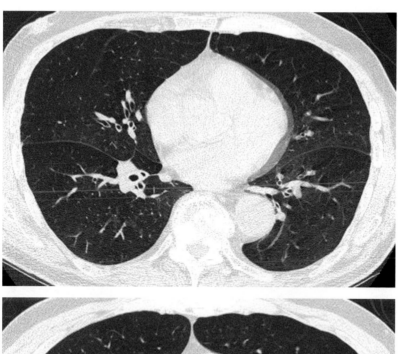

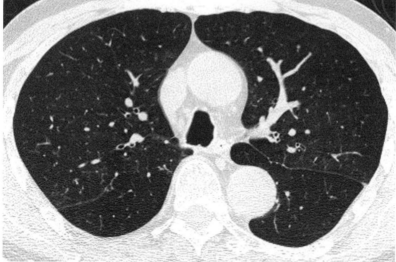

Fig. 4.1 HRCT chest.

Questions

4a) Describe the lung function test results.

4b) What do the CT images show?

4c) What investigations would you like to do next?

Answers

4a) **Describe the lung function test results.**

Fixed airflow obstruction with reduced diffusion capacity and transfer factor.

4b) **What do the CT images show?**

A typical 'tree-in-bud' appearance (arrow on close up view below) is seen characterized by small centrilobar soft tissue nodules connected by a branching linear opacity—this represents underlying bronchiolitis (normal

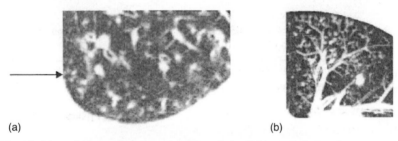

(a)　　　　　　　　　　　　　　　　　(b)

Fig. 4.2 (a) particularly good example of 'tree-in-bud' from another patient, (b) accentuated through a technique called 'maximum intensity projection.

'healthy' bronchioles are too small to be visible on CT). The distribution is predominantly sub-pleural. There is also some dilatation and bronchial wall thickening.

Table 4.2 Causes of tree-in-bud appearances on CT chest

Causal mechanism	Examples
Infection	Bacterial: *Staphylococcus aureus, Haemophilus influenzae*
	Mycobacterium tuberculosis, non-tuberculous *mycobacteria*
	Fungal
	Viral, e.g. *Cytomegalovirus, RSV*
Congenital disorder	Cystic fibrosis
Idiopathic	Obliterative bronchiolitis, diffuse panbronchiolitis (DPB)
Inhalation	Aspiration, toxic fumes
Connective tissue disease	Rheumatoid arthritis
Malignancy	Gastric/renal/breast, post-haematopoietic stem cell transplant

Pathologically the 'tree-in-bud' appearance correlates with intra-luminal exudate within peripheral airways and bronchiolar wall inflammation (bronchiolitis). There are multiple causes summarized in Table 4.2.

4c) **What investigations would you like to do next?**

- Routine blood tests, including differential white cell count
- Immunoglobulins, autoimmune profile
- Sputum analysis, culture and sensitivity (including three samples for AAFB analysis).

Investigations

- Hb 12.2g/dL, MCV 95.0fL, WCC 6.0×10^9/L (normal differential), platelets 348 x 10^9/L
- U&Es, LFTs and coagulation tests were normal
- CRP 12mg/L, ESR 24mm/h
- Immunoglobulins normal
- Rheumatoid factor negative
- Sputum, profuse growth of *Haemophilus influenzae*.

Progress

Despite 10-day courses of amoxicillin, erythromycin and cefuroxime, her cough persisted and repeat sputum cultures grew profuse amounts of *Haemophilus influenzae*.

Question

4d) What would you do next?

Answer

4d) **What would you do next?**

A prolonged course (e.g. at least 2 months) of an antibiotic to which the organism is susceptible would be a reasonable next step.

In this case, given the recent drug history and poor response to conventional antibiotic doses, a longer course of low-dose macrolide therapy could be prescribed, based on a recent European study (Poletti *et al.* 2003). This study described patients with similar clinical and radiological findings, all of whom cultured *Haemophilus influenzae* in sputum or bronchoalveolar lavage specimens. The authors reported a good response to low-dose macrolides and suggested that this cohort may represent a *forme fruste* of diffuse panbronchiolitis (see below) within a Caucasian population.

Progress

Shortly after starting clarithromycin, the cough resolved and spirometry returned to normal. Three months of therapy was completed and three years later she remains asymptomatic and off all medication.

Summary

Although bronchiolitis as a consequence of airway infection is recognized, the repeated isolation of *Haemophilus influenzae* in individuals with previously normal lung parenchyma is not widely reported. Its presence in patients with a productive cough and exertional dyspnoea should therefore alert physicians to the possibility of bronchiolitis either as (i) a precursor to, or a variant of, 'typical' diffuse panbronchiolitis (DPB) in a genetically distinct population, or (ii) as a consequence of refractory distal airways infection. These patients may benefit from a different therapeutic approach with a prolonged course of low-dose macrolides rather than repeated standard antimicrobial treatment.

Diffuse panbronchiolitis (DPB)

Diffuse panbronchiolitis (DPB) is a distinct form of small airways disease predominantly seen in Asian populations, particularly the Japanese. In contrast to *Haemophilus influenzae* related bronchiolitis, no causal factor has been identified although an infective aetiology is postulated. An association with HLA-Bw54 is seen, which is specific to East Asians, and is probably required for development of chronic sinus disease associated with DPB rather than the lung manifestations *per se*. This HLA type is uncommon in non-Orientals.

(In *Haemophilus influenzae* related bronchiolitis, the European *forme fruste* of DPB, sinus disease is less commonly found.) DPB is more prevalent in males and non-smokers in their 2nd to 5th decades. Death from progressive respiratory failure and cor pulmonale occurs without treatment.

Diagnostic criteria for DPB (Ministry of Health and Welfare of Japan)

- Productive cough (often >50mls sputum/day) and breathlessness
- History of chronic paranasal sinusitis
- Bilateral diffuse small nodular shadows on CXR or centrilobar micronodules on thoracic CT
- Coarse crackles
- FEV_1/FVC <70% and PaO_2 <80mmHg
- Titre of cold agglutinin ≥64.

Investigations

- 44% of cases culture *Haemophilus influenzae* in their sputum at presentation. *Pseudomonas* colonization increases with time (22% on presentation, 60% at four years)
- Cold agglutinins may be elevated in the absence of *Mycoplasma pneumoniae*
- Pulmonary function shows significant airflow obstruction with variable reduction in diffusing capacity
- HRCT findings are distinctive in DPB, but not pathognomonic, and the changes are graded:
  1. Nodules <5mm at end of bronchovascular branching structures
  2. 'Tree-in-bud' appearance
  3. Early bronchiectasis (cystic dilation of nodules)
  4. Large cysts and dilated proximal bronchi.

Management

Early macrolide treatment, e.g. oral erythromycin 400mg or 600mg daily (2nd line: clarithromycin 200–400mg or roxithromycin 150–300mg daily). The benefit of macrolides occurs at a minimum inhibitory concentration below that for an antibacterial effect and is supposed to be anti-inflammatory through inhibition of pro-inflammatory cytokines and suppression of neutrophil activity/ production.

Treatment should continue for at least 6 months to 2 years and cease when symptoms have improved with no ongoing functional limitation. Resolution of radiological abnormalities often correlates with clinical findings and even the most severe initial HRCT appearances can be expected to improve. The disappearance of centrilobar nodules from HRCT may also act as a surrogate indicator for timing the discontinuation of treatment. If symptoms persist, or return, then macrolide treatment should be restarted.

Prognosis

The prognosis of DPB was poor (33% survival at 10 years), but with use of macrolides it is now >90% at 10 years.

Further reading

Poletti V, Casoni G, Chilosi M, Zompatori M (2006). Diffuse panbronchiolitis. *Eur Respir J*; **28**: 862–871.

Case 5

A 51-year-old lady presented to A&E with shortness of breath for several months, much worse over the last 2 days, now with orthopnoea. Because of associated ankle swelling, she had been treated with diuretics 2 weeks earlier, which produced a 5kg weight loss and some temporary improvement in her shortness of breath. She had no associated history of chest pain, paroxysmal nocturnal dyspnoea, cough or sputum, no significant past medical history, and no personal or family history of lung disease. System review was negative. She had never smoked, was unemployed and had two children.

On examination:

- Tachypnoeic, undistressed, afebrile, obese (BMI, 40kg/m^2)
- Pulse 120 and regular, with respiratory paradox, BP 157/92mmHg, JVP to earlobes, 3rd heart sound
- Pitting oedema to thighs
- Crackles and wheezes in chest
- SaO_2 58% on air, 99% on high-flow oxygen
- ECG, sinus rhythm, small complexes and poor R wave progression.

A diagnosis of congestive cardiac failure, due to silent myocardial ischaemia, was made. She was given diuretics and O_2. Whilst awaiting a CXR, bloods and an echocardiogram were organized.

Investigations

- CXR, large heart, small bilateral pleural effusions, clear lung fields
- CRP, 134mg/L, WBC 12.4x10^9/L, U&Es normal
- Echocardiogram, small pericardial effusion, normal valves, good LV function, no ASD, right ventricle slightly dilated and hypertrophied, estimated peak pulmonary artery pressure of 60mmHg.

Five hours later she was semi-comatose and incontinent of urine. She was haemodynamically stable with a bounding pulse and warm peripheries, blood gases were done:

pH 7.16, PaO_2 32kPa, $PaCO_2$ 17.5kPa, base excess +10mmol/L.

Questions

5a) What is the evidence that she has been in ventilatory failure for a while?

5b) What is the most likely reason she became semi-comatose?

5c) Suggest some possible reasons for her ventilatory failure.

5d) Explain her fluid overload (cor pulmonale), why is this not 'right heart failure'?

Answers

5a) **What is the evidence that she has been in ventilatory failure for a while?**

She has a raised base excess (+10mmol/l), which indicates a metabolic alkalosis. This has presumably been caused by renal retention of bicarbonate to compensate for a chronically raised $PaCO_2$. Base excess values as high as this are very rarely caused by any other mechanism, such as diuretic therapy, hypokalaemia, or prolonged vomiting.

5b) **What is the most likely reason she became semi-comatose?**

The most likely reason for her semi-comatose state is the respiratory acidosis caused by the high $PaCO_2$, consequent on her having been given too high a concentration of oxygen in the presence of prior hypercapnic ventilatory failure.

5c) **Suggest some possible reasons for her ventilatory failure.**

Chronic ventilatory failure (and therefore sensitivity to excessive oxygen levels) can have many causes, but the more likely can be classified most simply as follows (*indicates the commonest causes):

- ◆ Primary failure of ventilatory drive—a brainstem abnormality, e.g. Arnold Chiari malformation, brainstem stroke, polio, and post-polio syndrome, syringobulbia, Ondine's curse (e.g. PHOX2B gene abnormalities)
- ◆ Pump failure due to a weak pump or 'bellows' function
  - *neuropathies, e.g. motor neurone disease (especially if diaphragm involved early), isolated bilateral diaphragm paralysis (e.g. brachial neuritis), spinal muscular atrophy, Guillain-Barré
  - *myopathies, e.g. acid maltase deficiency, (diaphragm usually involved early), Duchenne muscular dystrophy, myotonic dystrophy
  - neuromuscular junction, e.g. myasthenia gravis
- ◆ Pump failure due to a heavy load
  - *lower airways obstruction e.g. COPD, chronic asthma, bronchiolitis
  - *obstructive sleep apnoea (OSA, when with co-morbidities)
  - chest wall, e.g. *scoliosis, *obesity.

When a patient is found to be in unexpected ventilatory failure, in reality the commonest causes are indicated with an asterisk* above. There may well be more than one reason with, for example, a mixture of COPD, obesity and OSA all being present; in fact OSA rarely causes diurnal ventilatory failure on its own, but is a potent provoker when combined with

COPD and/or morbid obesity. Elucidation of the contributing cause(s) is clearly important before the correct therapy can be given.

5d) **Explain her fluid overload (cor pulmonale), why is this not 'right heart failure'?**

Cor pulmonale. Chronic hypoxia leads to salt and excessive water retention, probably through increased sympathetic drive to the kidney. Excess fluid is stored in the venous system, and thus leads to a raised JVP and dependant oedema (if there is left ventricular dysfunction as well, then pulmonary oedema may also result). In addition, there will be hypoxic pulmonary vasoconstriction with a gradual rise in pulmonary artery pressure and right ventricular hypertrophy, but *no evidence* of poor right ventricular function. There is no reduction in cardiac output; in fact there may be a rise due to the vasodilation caused by the raised $PaCO_2$ (which may also exacerbate movement of water across capillaries, thus exacerbating the oedema). Hence a common term for this situation, right heart failure, is incorrect: a raised JVP does not automatically mean there is right heart failure as it would, for instance, after a large pulmonary embolus or right sided myocardial infarction.

Further progress

The patient was resuscitated with non-invasive ventilation administered via a face mask and rapidly regained consciousness. Repeat history revealed no symptoms of muscle weakness or of brachial neuritis (also called neuralgic amyotrophy), where there can be variable involvement of the brachial plexus nerves (including phrenic nerves) with shoulder pain and sometime scapular winging (aetiology unknown). There was no history of snoring or witnessed apnoeas, although there had been recent sleepiness. The family confirmed that she had never smoked. Re-examination did not suggest diaphragm weakness (no abdominal paradox during inspiration or sniffing). There was no fasciculation to suggest motor neurone disease. CT scan of the lungs was normal apart from evidence of air trapping.

Lung function

See Table 5.1.

Table 5.1 Pulmonary function tests

	Measured	Predicted normal	Post salbutamol
FEV_1(L)	0.5	2.4	0.9
VC (L)	1.8	3.0	2.2
FEV_1/VC (%)	30	75	41
FRC(L)	4.2	2.6	
RV(L)	3.5	1.7	
TLC(L)	6.5	4.6	
RAW(kPa/L/s)	0.53	<0.2	
K_{CO}(mmol/min/kPa/L)	1.51	1.66	

Flow volume loops showed no evidence of upper airways obstruction

Questions

5e) What do the lung function tests show?

5f) What is the likely diagnosis?

5g) Suggest the most useful therapeutic trial.

Answers

5e) **What do the lung function test show?**

The lung function tests show severe airways obstruction with marked air trapping. There is significant reversibility.

5f) **What is the likely diagnosis?**

This pattern would be compatible with asthma, COPD or bronchiolitis; however, the improved FEV_1, and reduced air trapping (increased VC), following bronchodilators would most favour asthma. The increased TLC would more favour emphysema, but the normal K_{CO} would not.

5g) **Suggest the most useful therapeutic trial.**

A trial of steroids would identify if the airways obstruction was due to asthma, or possibly bronchiolitis, and define the full extent of its reversibility.

Further progress

A trial of steroids led to a gradual improvement in lung function and, surprisingly, a virtual return to normal values. Blood gases returned to normal with resolution of all signs of cor pulmonale. This improvement was maintained with inhaled steroids and long-acting bronchodilators. An assumed diagnosis of chronic asthma was made and, in retrospect, had been present for some months prior to presentation to A&E.

It is very unusual for asthma to present in this way, mimicking the airways obstruction, ventilatory failure, and cor pulmonale that is most often due to smoking-induced COPD. Presumably she had a relatively low hypoxic ventilatory drive, which, along with significant obesity (BMI about 40), allowed this unusual presentation with hypercapnia. Large variations in hypoxic ventilatory drives are seen within normal populations.

Further reading

Chapman S, Robinson G, Stradling J and West S (2009). *Oxford Handbook of Respiratory Medicine*, 2nd edn, chapter 15 and 23, p. 91 and 201.

Case 6

Case A

A 54-year-old Asian man presented to the emergency department with a 3-month history of increasing dyspnoea, drenching night sweats and weight loss. This was associated with a dry cough and occasional small volume haemoptysis. He was born in Pakistan, moved to the UK 3 years previously and had visited his family in Pakistan 4 months previously. He worked in a restaurant and smoked 20 cigarettes per day.

On examination, there was cervical lymphadenopathy and signs of a left pleural effusion. A chest drain was inserted and the effusion drained to dryness.

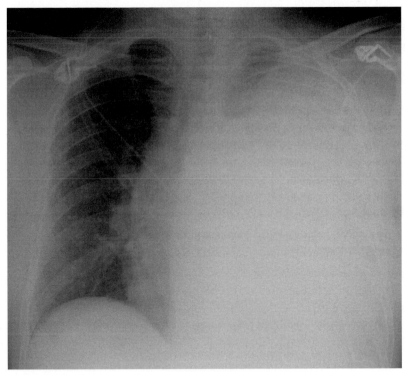

Fig. 6.1 CXR (case A).

Blood results:

- Hb, 10.7g/dL
- WCC, 14.3 × 10⁹/L
- CRP, 40mg/l
- Electrolytes normal
- Mildly raised Alk phos (275IU/L)
- Other LFTs normal
- Tuberculin skin test, grade II positive
- Sputum, smear negative for AAFBs, blood-stained.

Pleural fluid results:

- Protein 43g/dL
- Glucose 5.2mmol/L
- LDH 416 IU/L (normal 150–220)
- 30% lymphocytes
- No bacteria, no mycobacteria on ZN stain.

He was started on anti-tuberculosis chemotherapy (rifampicin, isoniazid, pyrazinamide, ethambutol) pending sputum TB cultures. Four weeks later he was referred to the respiratory department with persistent symptoms and worsening liver function tests (alk phos = 350IU/L, ALT =120IU/L, normal bilirubin). TB cultures were still pending.

Case B

A 19-year-old Chinese man was referred to the respiratory department with a 3-month history of increasing right-sided chest pain, and a 1-week history of vomiting. He remained physically very active with a minor decrease in his exercise ability only. He had moved from China to the UK at the age of 12. CXR revealed a large right-sided pleural effusion. He had visited his parents in China 1 month previously and had been started on 3 agent TB treatment by a local doctor (rifampicin, isoniazid, pyrazinamide), with which he was continuing, despite the vomiting.

Investigations showed raised inflammatory markers (WCC = 15 × 10⁹/L, CRP = 58mg/L) and anaemia (Hb = 8.7g/dL). Other blood tests were normal. Tuberculin skin test was grade II positive, and pleural fluid results as follows:

- Blood-stained fluid
- Protein 39g/dL

- Glucose 4.1mmol/L
- LDH 617IU/L (normal 150–220)
- 40% lymphocytes
- No bacteria, no mycobacteria on ZN stains
- Sputum cultures: pending.

Questions

6a) How would you now manage the anti-tuberculosis medications in each of these cases?

6b) Are any further investigations required in each case; if so, which and why?

Answers

6a) **How would you now manage the anti-tuberculosis medications in each of these cases?**

Both of these patients have symptoms or investigations that may be consistent with side-effects of anti-tuberculosis therapy (deranged LFTs in case A, and vomiting in case B). However, some thought should be given to the confidence of the diagnosis of TB, especially in the presence of apparent treatment side-effects.

In neither case is there a definitive microbiological diagnosis. Although the tuberculin skin test is mildly positive, this would be an unusual result in a patient with active TB (one would expect either no response due to immune suppression, or florid positivity). In addition, the pleural fluid characteristics are against TB pleuritis (in which one would expect a low-normal glucose and lymphocyte predominance—see Case 13) and TB effusions are not usually blood-stained. Both patients are anaemic, which is a common finding in TB; however, in the presence of TB pleuritis alone (an immunological reaction to MTB within the pleural space) this is unusual.

Given the insecure diagnosis, and possible treatment complications in both these cases, TB treatment should be stopped until a firm diagnosis is established. If all medications are halted at the same time, there is little chance of resistant organisms developing.

6b) **Are any further investigations required in each case; if so, which and why?**

Further investigations are required to establish the diagnosis firmly as above. Investigations to consider are:

- Further imaging—thoracic CT scan with contrast would be helpful in delineating any pleural abnormality, and may reveal parenchymal disease consistent with TB, allowing direction of further investigations (e.g. bronchoscopy). The scan should be performed with some pleural fluid left in situ to improve pleural tissue contrast (i.e. not drained to dryness).

- Obtain pleural tissue—'blind' (i.e. non-image guided, e.g. Abram's) pleural biopsy has a good sensitivity (overall around 80%) in the case of pleural TB. Thoracoscopy and CT-guided biopsy have a higher sensitivity than this and are the investigations of choice, if other diagnoses (e.g. malignancy) are in the differential.

- Immunological tests for TB (e.g. interferon gamma assays—see Case 31). While these tests are highly sensitive in the diagnosis of latent TB, there is controversy as to their role in the diagnosis of active TB infection. Even if the test is strongly positive, no microbiological information and sensitivities to anti-tuberculosis drugs are available.

Progress

Pleural TB was not considered to be a likely diagnosis in either of these two cases for the reasons given above. Both patients went on to have thoracic CT with contrast enhancement, which are shown in Fig. 6.2.

Case A

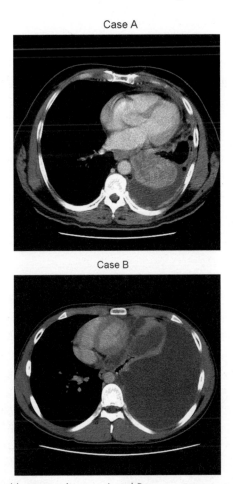

Case B

Fig. 6.2 CT chest with contrast in cases A and B.

Questions

6c) Interpret the CT images.

6d) What is now the most likely diagnosis in each case, and how would you investigate these patients further?

Answers

6c) **Interpret the CT images.**

Case A

There is a pleural effusion associated with nodular irregular areas of pleural thickening, with areas of air within the fluid (indicating loculations and presumed secondary to previous drainage). The atelectatic lung appears to contain areas of low attenuation, raising the suspicion of a lesion within the lower lobe.

Case B

There is a large left effusion with areas of enhancement in the posterior thorax. In addition, there is a separate area anteriorly abutting the pericardium that could represent a locule (with a wide septation separating it from the rest of the pleural fluid) or a cystic mass.

6d) **What is now the most likely diagnosis in each case, and how would you investigate these patients further?**

In Case A, this is now most likely to represent malignant pleural disease, and is likely to be a lung primary with spread to the pleura (staging it as

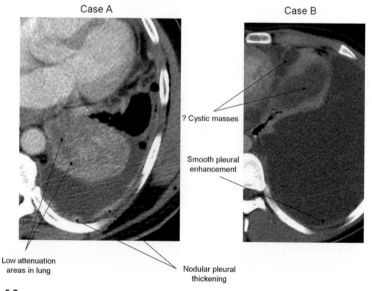

Fig. 6.3

T4 disease under the current TNM classification, in the absence of information on nodal involvement and distant metastases). Pleural biopsy (by thoracoscopy or CT guidance) is the next best test to achieve a diagnosis.

In Case B, the likely diagnosis will depend on further characterization of the possible cystic mass seen in the anterior thorax. If this area represents highly septated pleural fluid, the differential remains wide (pleural infection, inflammatory disorders, longstanding transudates, malignancy). If, however, a cystic mass is identified, malignancy (e.g. germ cell tumour in this age group) becomes more likely. The easiest next investigation may therefore be an ultrasound to characterize the anterior lesion, or an MRI. Given the young age of this patient, and the extent of the disease, he underwent a video-assisted thoracoscopic (VATs) procedure, to achieve accurate macroscopic and histological diagnosis, and to clear the pleural space of fluid and septations.

Progress

Case A

The patient underwent local anaesthetic thoracoscopy, which revealed macroscopic evidence of pleural malignancy. Multiple biopsies were taken and a talc pleurodesis performed to prevent fluid recurrence. The biopsies showed adenocarcinoma of likely lung origin, which was considered inoperable (stage IIIb disease), and he therefore proceeded to palliative chemotherapy and survived only a few months.

Case B

Ultrasound was suggestive of a mass lesion rather than septated fluid in the area abutting the pericardium. The patient underwent VATs, which revealed a cystic mass lesion. Multiple biopsies were taken, and the septated effusion cleared. Biopsies revealed abnormal cells with spindle cell morphology, consistent with a sarcoma. He went on to receive chemotherapy, and died 7 months later.

Case 7

A 32-year-old American woman was referred for investigation of left-sided subcostal pleuritic chest pain. Four months earlier she had been treated for left lower lobe pneumonia (radiologically confirmed) requiring two courses of antibiotics (amoxicillin and erythromycin). After this illness the chest pain persisted, and she felt 'tired and drained'. She also reported an intermittent cough, productive of small amounts of 'off-white' sputum, but denied other respiratory symptoms. She had had no haemoptysis, fevers or sweats, anorexia or weight loss. She had a history of a left-sided pneumonia aged 8, and of being 'chesty' until 13; otherwise she had been well. She had never smoked, and seldom drank alcohol. There were no abnormal physical signs. Her CXRs are shown in Fig. 7.1a and b.

Questions

7a) What do the CXRs show?

7b) List potential causes for the ongoing symptoms?

7c) What investigation would you like to do next?

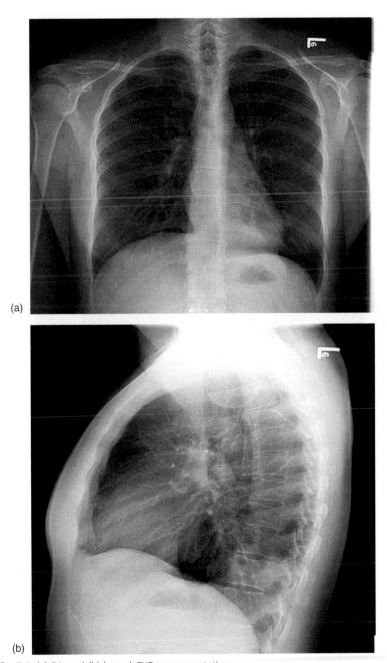

Fig. 7.1 (a) PA and (b) lateral CXR on presentation.

Answers

7a) What do the CXRs show?

Consolidation is seen within the postero-basal segment of the left lower lobe (retro-cardiac opacification) on both the PA and lateral images (see Fig. 7.2).

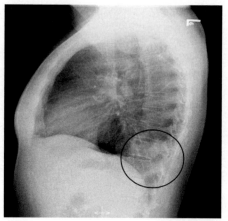

Fig. 7.2 Lateral CXR: retro-cardiac area of consolidation circled.

7b) List potential causes for the ongoing symptoms?

Potential causes for this patient's ongoing pleuritic chest pain, intermittent productive cough and radiological non-resolution could be:

Common:

◆ Infection

• Post-infectious pleurisy usually recedes quickly with antibiotic therapy supplemented with appropriate analgesia. Prolonged post-infective cough is common (especially with viral aetiologies) and can last for months.

• Ongoing symptoms and non-radiological resolution, following standard anti-microbial therapy, should raise suspicion of atypical pathogens, e.g. *Legionella* spp., *Mycoplasma*, *Chlamydia pneumoniae*, fungi or mycobacteria

◆ Malignancy

- Suppurative lung disease
  - Underlying bronchiectasis or a lung abscess should be considered although the radiological appearances are not typical for the latter.

Less common:

- Recurrent gastric aspiration
- Thromboembolic disease (with resultant infarction accounting for the radiological change)
- Cryptogenic organizing pneumonia (COP)
- Eosinophilic lung disease, e.g. eosinophilic pneumonia or allergic bronchopulmonary aspergillosis (ABPA, usually upper lobe predominant)
- Vasculitis/collagen vascular disease, such as Wegener's granulomatosis or rheumatoid arthritis
- Congenital abnormality, e.g. bronchogenic cyst, bronchopulmonary sequestration
- Drug-induced lung disease.

7c) **What investigation would you like to do next?**

Contrast-enhanced thoracic CT would be a suitable next investigation in view of the failure of clinical improvement and lack of radiological resolution 8 weeks following appropriate therapy.

Further information

She had no history of chronic chest disease, tuberculosis, collagen vascular disease, radiation exposure, foreign body inhalation or risk factors for acquired immunodeficiency states.

Investigations

- Hb 15.2g/dL, MCV 86.5fL, WCC 9.2×10^9/L (normal differential), platelets 387×10^9/L
- U&E, LFT, glucose, TFT all normal
- CRP <8mg/L, ESR 10mm/h
- Immunoglobulins, normal
- Antinuclear antibodies and rheumatoid factor, negative

- *Streptococcus pneumoniae* and *Haemophilus influenzae* antibody responses within the normal range
- Sputum culture, no growth
- Full pulmonary function tests, normal.
- Contrast enhanced thoracic CT scan (Fig. 7.3).

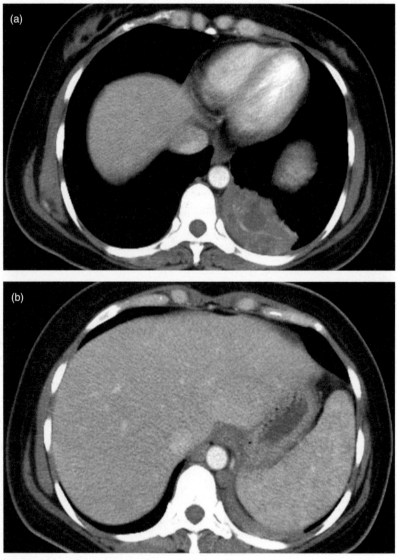

Fig. 7.3 (a) and (b) Contrast-enhanced CT chest images.

Questions

7d) What does the CT scan demonstrate?

7e) What is the diagnosis?

7f) What are the treatment options?

Answers

7d) What does the CT scan demonstrate?

The magnified CT image in Fig. 7.4a demonstrates heterogeneous consolidation within the left base sharing an irregular border with the neighbouring lung parenchyma. Cystic components are evident and an anomalous vessel is present within the mass (arrow).

In the CT (Fig. 7.4b), this vessel can be seen as it originates from the aorta (arrow) and (images not shown) leads directly into the lesion. The lungs are otherwise normal.

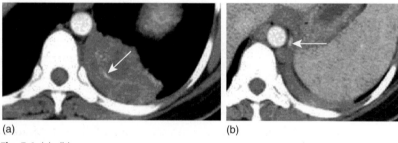

(a)   (b)

Fig. 7.4 (a), (b)

7e) What is the diagnosis?

These findings are in keeping with a diagnosis of intralobar sequestration (ILS).

Pulmonary sequestration is rare and accounts for 0.15–6.4% of all congenital pulmonary malformations. It is characterized by the presence of a segment of lung that has no identifiable contact with the normal bronchial tree and derives its blood supply from an anomalous systemic artery. Two types are recognized: intralobar (ILS) and extralobar sequestration (ELS). Table 7.1 summarizes the main clinical differences.

- ◆ Other congenital anomalies (e.g. diaphragmatic hernias, congenital cystic adenomatoid malformation type (CCAM) II and cardiopulmonary disease) are seen in 10–14% of those with intralobar and 50% of those with extralobar sequestration.

- ◆ The exact aetiology of pulmonary sequestration is unknown.
  - Development of ELS from an accessory lung bud, which arises caudally from primitive foregut, is postulated. It is theorized that this

Table 7.1

	Intralobar sequestration	Extralobar sequestration
Frequency	75%	25%
Appearance	Within visceral pleura of the normal lung	Enclosed in a separate pleural sac
Sex ratio	1M:1F	4M:1F
Site	98% lower lobe 60% left-sided	95% left-sided 75% within costophrenic angle 10–15% sub-diaphragmatic
Presentation	Rare <2 years, often history of recurrent pneumonia in adulthood	61% at <6 months
Asymptomatic cases (incidental finding)	15%	10%

segment retains splanchnic (systemic) blood supply generating traction on the lung fragment, which subsequently segregates from the main lung mass.

- The origin of ILS is contentious. The 'congenital' hypothesis mirrors that of ELS formation, whereas in the 'acquired' theory, ILS arises from transformation of chronically inflamed normal lung (pseudosequestration), i.e. the presence of an obstructed bronchus (mediated by inflammation, aspiration or infection) causing secondary occlusion of the local pulmonary artery supply leading to systemic arterial parasitisation with vessel incorporation into the, now sequestered, pulmonary tissue.

- Patients often present with cough +/– sputum production, recurrent pneumonia or features secondary to related anomalies. Superimposed infections, i.e. fungal, tuberculosis, massive haemoptysis, haemothorax and cardiovascular complications can occur. Benign and malignant tumours have been reported arising in sequestered lung.

- Chest radiography typically shows lower lobe homogeneous consolidation or a mass. Cavitation and cystic areas may occur.

- CT allows further definition of areas of sequestration. ILS characteristically manifests as a homogeneous or heterogeneous mass sharing an irregular border with adjacent lung. Cavities may be seen and cysts with air-fluid levels present. The aberrant vessel supplying the lesion is visualized in up to 80% of cases. Other associated anomalies may be noted.

- Conventional angiography has been the gold standard for abnormal vascular connections however non-invasive CT angiography and magnetic resonance angiography are now superseding its use.

7f) **What are the treatment options?**

Treatment options:

- Symptomatic pulmonary sequestration: surgical resection, once infection has subsided, is recommended and can usually be performed thoracoscopically (VATs)
  - Lobectomy is commonly performed for ILS
  - Sequestrectomy for ELS cases is the usual approach
- Pre-operative identification of aberrant vessels is helpful but is not a pre-requisite of successful surgery
- The management of asymptomatic pulmonary sequestration is controversial, with some advocating routine resection and others opting for a conservative non-operative approach.

Prognosis is good, and resection of the abnormal segment is usually curative. Any mortality often reflects the presence of accompanying anomalies.

Progress

The patient remained well with only occasional low grade left-sided chest pain. She opted against surgical resection, but was advised to take antibiotics promptly if she developed infective symptoms.

Further reading

Corbett HJ, Humphrey GME (2004). Pulmonary sequestration. *Paediatric Respiratory Reviews*; **5**: 59–68.

Frazier AA, Rosado de Christenson MI, Stoker JT, Templeton PA (1997). Intralobar sequestration: radiologic-pathologic correlation. *Radiographics*; **17**: 725–745.

Case 8

A 40-year-old accountant, recently moved into the area, presented with a 3-month history of cough and, over the previous month, dyspnoea on exercise. Initially antibiotics seemed to help, although repeated sputum cultures were negative. Whilst skiing at 3000m, he developed severe dyspnoea, which greatly curtailed his physical activity. On his return he also noticed some dyspnoea during his usual exercise of cycling and circuit training.

He had no relevant past medical history, apart from mild hayfever as a teenager. He had never smoked, drank six units of alcohol a week, and had no pets. He was married, heterosexual, with only one partner for many years. There was no history of reflux, sinusitis or wheeze.

On examination

On auscultation there were obvious fine bi-basal end-inspiratory crackles. His resting arterial oxygen saturation was 97% on air, but fell to 93% after 30 steps up and down a 9in-high block.

Investigations

- CXR, equivocal diffuse shadowing throughout
- FBC, U&Es and liver function tests were all normal
- ANA/ANCA, negative; rheumatoid factor, 1/80; ESR, 14mm/h; CRP, 60mg/L
- Serology, Q fever, psittacosis, mycoplasma, influenza A&B, legionella: all negative
- Proteins and electrophoresis, IgG 22.5g/L (upper limit 13.0g/L), otherwise normal
- Budgerigar, pigeon and hen precipitins, negative
- Pulmonary function, Table 8.1.

Table 8.1 Pulmonary function tests

	Measured	Predicted
FEV_1(L)	3.2	3.3
VC (L)	3.7	4.0
FEV_1/VC%	86	75–85%
VA(L)	5.5	5.9
TL_{CO}(mmol/min/kPa)	7.6	9.2
K_{CO}(mmol/min/kPa/L)	1.39	1.70

Questions

8a) Suggest the two most likely diagnostic categories.

8b) Would you expect this drop of 4% SaO_2 on exercise in a normal person?

8c) Are the lung function results abnormal?

8d) What would be the most useful next investigation?

Answers

8a) **Suggest the two most likely diagnostic categories.**

The raised CRP, raised IgG and initial response to antibiotics, would suggest possible infection, but the history is a little long for this to be the likely explanation of all the symptoms. The CXR may indicate a viral infection, but is more likely to be due to a diffuse interstitial pneumonitis. The presence of crackles virtually rules out sarcoidosis, but still leaves a wide differential.

8b) **Would you expect this drop of 4% SaO$_2$ on exercise in a normal person?**

The SaO$_2$ should not drop, even on heavy exercise, with a normal heart and lungs at sea level. A drop from 97% to 93% is equivalent to a fall in PaO$_2$ of 3.3kPa, and is clearly abnormal. However, it is important to do this test properly. Oximeters work by measuring the two relevant wavelengths (registering oxygenated and total haemoglobin) in pulsatile blood only, hence responding only to arterial blood and disregarding non-pulsatile capillary and venous blood. If the hand is moving during the exercise, this can make the venous blood pulsate, thus fooling the oximeter into registering venous as well as arterial blood (particularly if the cardiac output is low) and giving a falsely low value. Thus the reading is best taken when the patient has sat down after exercise, and the hand has been still for 15–30 seconds (this is well before the SaO$_2$ begins to recover after exercise).

8c) **Are the lung function results abnormal?**

The lung function is technically within the normal range but, given the overall scenario, the fact that the gas transfer is towards the bottom end of normal in a previously fit individual is supportive of interstitial lung disease.

8d) **What would be the most useful next investgation?**

A high resolution CT scan (HRCT) will be the next most useful test, differentiating between many of the different interstitial lung diseases.

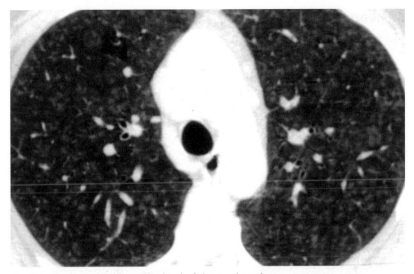

Fig. 8.1 Single HRCT slice at the level of the aortic arch.

Questions

8e) What does the HRCT slice in Fig. 8.1 show?

8f) What should be done next to try and make a diagnosis?

Answers

8e) What does the HRCT slice in Fig. 8.1 show?

The HRCT appearances are typical of hypersensitivity pneumonitis (or extrinsic allergic alveolitis, Fig. 8.2a). Multiple poorly-defined nodules are seen centred around the middle of the secondary pulmonary lobule (Fig. 8.2b), centrilobar or peribronchial (i.e. at the bronchovascular bundle where the main antibody/antigen reaction occurs).

8f) What should be done next to try and make a diagnosis?

The history should be revisited—was exposure to a relevant allergen missed? Lung biopsy could be considered for histological confirmation.

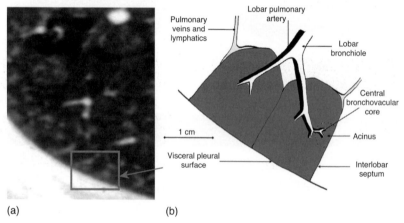

(a)   (b)

Fig. 8.2 (a) Actual and (b) schematic depiction of secondary pulmonary lobule.

Progress

Repeat history revealed that 6 months before presentation he had moved into an old thatched cottage. Symptoms had begun a few months later. Sometimes the antigen responsible cannot be identified, but this story raises the possibility of a fungus being responsible. *Aspergillus* precipitins were negative and therefore further fungi were tested on agar diffusion (Ouchterlony) plates.

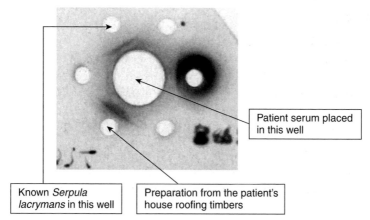

Patient serum placed in this well

Known *Serpula lacrymans* in this well

Preparation from the patient's house roofing timbers

Fig. 8.3 Ouchterlony results.

Questions

8g) What does the Ouchterlony plate in Fig. 8.3 show?

8h) What is the cause?

8i) What is the treatment?

Answers

8g) **What does the Ouchterlony plate in Fig. 8.3 show?**

Precipitin lines have formed where antigen (peripheral wells) meets precipitating antibody (central well) (Fig. 8.3). More detailed analysis showed there was more than one line, indicating that the patient was making IgG to more than one epitope on *Serpula lacrymans*. The number of lines is roughly proportional to the degree of immunological reaction to the fungus.

8h) **What is the cause?**

Serpula lacrymans is the main fungus causing dry rot. It is called lacrymans, not because you cry when you find it in your house, but because water drops often form on the fungus, like tears (Fig. 8.4).

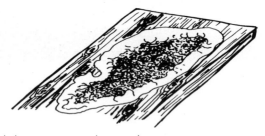

Fig. 8.4 *Serpula lacrymans* on rotting wood.

8i) **What is the treatment?**

Hypersensitivity pneumonitis (histology shown in Fig 8.5) responds well to steroids with rapid relief of symptoms, as occurred in this case. Once the dry rot had been identified in the roof, the patient sold his cottage as quickly as possible, thus removing himself from the antigen.

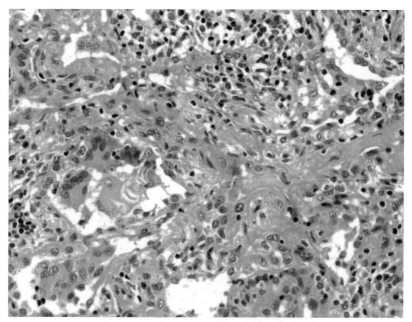

Fig. 8.5 Lung biopsy showing small, poorly-formed non-caseating granulomas, located near respiratory or terminal bronchioles (courtesy of Dr C. Clelland).

With thanks to Prof Rob Davies for permission to report this case, and to Dr Graham Bird (deceased), who first recognized that dry rot was the explanation.

Further reading

Bryant DH, Rogers P (1991). Allergic alveolitis due to wood-rot fungi. *Allergy Proc*; **12**: 89–94.

Case 9

An 18-year-old student had bilateral pneumothoraces, which had not resolved with simple aspiration and chest drain insertion. She therefore underwent bilateral pleurectomy, during which it was observed she had multiple small cysts over the surfaces of her lungs. She made a good recovery, although was left with a chronic left pneumothorax. Histology of a lung biopsy at the time of surgery is shown in Fig. 9.1, and her CXR and CT chest in Fig. 9.2a and b. She had never smoked, and her only past medical history was of a renal angiomyolipoma, for which she underwent a left nephrectomy aged 13.

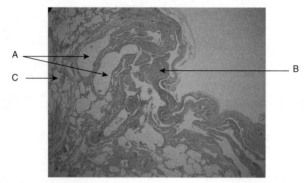

Fig. 9.1 Histology of lung biopsy, taken at the time of surgery, with H&E stain. Features A to C are referred to in Answer 9a.

Questions

9a) What features are illustrated in Figs 9.1 and 9.2?

9b) What conditions cause pulmonary cysts, and what radiological features distinguish them?

9c) What is the most likely diagnosis?

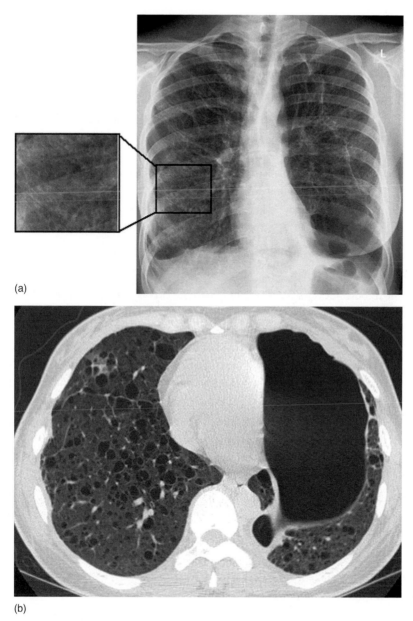

(a)

(b)

Fig. 9.2 (a) CXR and (b) CT chest.

Answers

9a) **What features are illustrated in Figs. 9.1 and 9.2?**

Histology (Fig. 9.1) shows the presence of cysts (see label A), and areas of focal smooth muscle proliferation (B). Alveoli with distorted architecture are seen to the left of the image, probably crush artifact (C).

The CXR (Fig. 9.2a) shows a left-sided pneumothorax, with lucency at the left base, and the lung edge visible up to the left apex. There is apparent interstitial shadowing without thoracic volume loss (e.g. see enlarged portion). Interstitial shadowing on a CXR is often due to fibrosis, and so associated with volume loss. Interstitial shadowing without volume loss is unusual, and should make one think of these three conditions:

- Lymphangioleiomyomatosis (LAM)
- Langerhans cell histiocytosis (LCH, or histiocytosis X)
- Lymphangitiis.

In both LAM and LCH the lung parenchyma is essentially normal; however, the presence of multiple cysts gives the false impression on plain CXR of interstitial shadowing and reticulae (lines). As there is normal parenchyma, lung volumes are not reduced, as they would be in fibrotic conditions. In pure lymphangitiis, again the parenchyma is normal, but malignant spread through pulmonary lymphatics produces interstitial shadowing on the CXR.

The HRCT chest (Fig. 9.2b) shows the left pneumothorax, and multiple small thin-walled cysts scattered evenly throughout the lung fields. This widespread distribution is typical of LAM. The intervening lung parenchyma appears normal.

9b) **What conditions cause pulmonary cysts, and what radiological features distinguish them?**

Pulmonary cysts may arise in:

- Lymphangioleiomyomatosis (LAM)
- Langerhans cell histiocytosis (LCH)
- End stage pulmonary fibrosis with honeycombing.

Cysts are round spaces with well-defined walls, which are usually air-containing when in the lung, though may also contain fluid. Their walls are made up of respiratory epithelium, cartilage or smooth muscle. In contrast, bullae are usually present in emphysema. These are air-filled spaces, with thin walls (<1mm) made up of pleura, septa or compressed

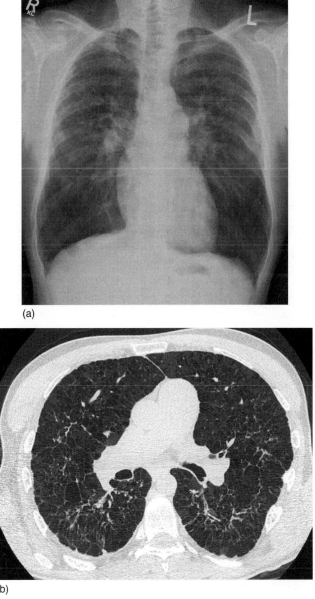

Fig. 9.3 (a) CXR and (b) HRCT chest of a patient with Langerhans cell histiocytosis. This rare granulomatous condition is associated with smoking. It has a mid- and upper-zone predominance, whereas LAM affects all zones equally. Characteristic features of the CT scan are 'bizarre' or irregular-shaped cysts and nodules. In LAM cysts are regular, and nodules are not present.

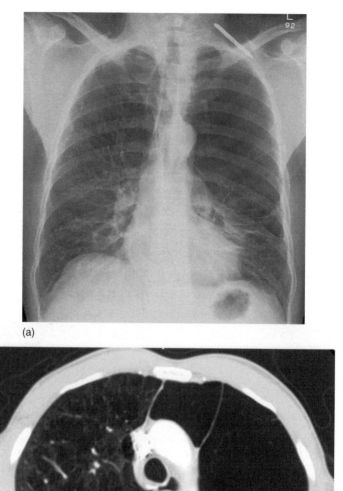

(a)

(b)

Fig. 9.4 (a) CXR and (b) CT chest of a patient with severe COPD with bullous lung disease. On the CXR there is a focal region of low attenuation in the left mid-zone, without visible walls, due to a massively enlarged air space. On CT scan, bullae are large and irregular, with no or thin walls. The bullae often have a central vessel, distinguishing them from cysts.

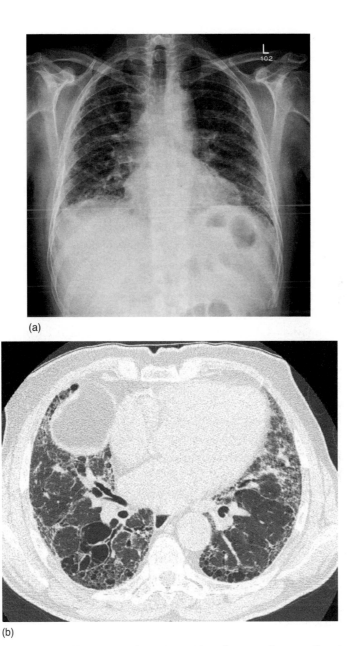

(a)

(b)

Fig. 9.5 (a) CXR and (b) CT chest of a patient with end-stage pulmonary fibrosis secondary to usual interstitial pneumonitis (UIP). The chest XR shows markedly reduced thoracic volumes. The cysts on the CT are peripheral and thick walled.

lung tissue. Distinguishing radiological features of LCH, emphysema and fibrosis are highlighted below (Figs 9.3, 9.4 and 9.5).

9c) **What is the most likely diagnosis?**

Lymphangioleiomyomatosis (LAM) dyspnoea, multiple pneumothoraces, the previous history of an angiomyolipoma and characteristic CT changes are all highly suggestive of LAM. In such cases it is not essential to obtain a histological diagnosis.

LAM is a rare condition in which abnormal smooth muscle cells progressively accumulate in the lungs and lymphatics. Abnormalities in the proteins tuberin and hamartin (which usually attenuate smooth muscle growth), are found within LAM tissue. It has a prevalence in sporadic cases of 1 in 1,000,000. It is much more common in patients with the genetic disease tuberous sclerosis, where signs of LAM can be identified in up to 40% of adult females. It almost exclusively affects females, generally developing between menarche and the menopause, with a mean age of onset in the mid-30s. The first symptom in most patients is either dyspnoea or pneumothorax. Less common presentations are cough, haemoptysis or chylous pleural effusions. Occasionally abdominal symptoms and signs precede respiratory symptoms. Physical examination is often normal early in the disease unless a pneumothorax or chylous effusion is present, although a minority of patients have crackles and wheeze. Other CT features of LAM besides those illustrated above are angiomyolipomas (consisting of fat, smooth muscle and thick walled blood vessels), lymphangioleiomyomas (proliferation of smooth muscle cells in lymph vessels causing collections of chylous fluid) and chylous pleural or ascitic collections. Survival in LAM is around 70% at 10 years, although this is highly variable. All patients with LAM should undergo evaluation for stigmata of tuberous sclerosis since these conditions often co-exist, with tuberous sclerosis occurring in 15% of women with LAM. These include periungual fibromas, facial angiofibromas, Shagreen patches (yellowish-pink firm skin plaques with a pebble-like texture) and hypomelanotic patches.

Progress report

Over the next 4 years she remained stable, with a chronic left pneumothorax, and only mild exercise limitation. She was keen to fly in order to see her parents who live overseas. Her CXR showed no progressive changes. Full pulmonary function tests were carried out (Table 9.1).

Table 9.1 Pulmonary function tests

	Measured
SaO_2(%)	97
FEV_1(L)	1.6 (53% pred)
FVC(L)	2.0 (56% pred)
FEV_1/FVC ratio	78%
FRC(L)	3.2 (120% pred) body plethysmographic method
RV(L)	2.4 (190% pred) body plethysmographic method
TLC(L)	4.5 (99% pred) body plethysmographic method
	3.0 (67% pred) helium dilution method
TL_{CO}(mM/min/kPa)	4.99 (51% pred)
K_{CO}(mM/min/kPa/L)	1.86 (86% pred)

Questions

9d) Describe the pulmonary function tests. What is the estimated size of the trapped, non-communicating air (this includes the pneumothoraces and cysts)? What other method might help quantify the size of a pneumothorax?

9e) What is the theoretical risk of flying, and how would she conventionally be advised?

Answers

9d) **Describe the pulmonary function tests. What is the estimated size of the trapped, non-communicating air (this includes the pneumothoraces and cysts)? What other method might help quantify the size of a pneumothorax?**

In this case, pulmonary function tests show a restrictive defect, with proportionate reduction in FEV_1 and FVC. This is likely to be due to her pneumothorax. In many patients, airflow obstruction predominates potentially leading to a mis-diagnosis of COPD.

The two methods of measuring TLC give different values. Body plethysmography measures total volume within the thorax, whereas helium dilution only measures gas in communication with the airways within the time of the 10-second breath hold, thus excluding gas in pneumothoraces and cysts. The difference between the two gives the size of the non-communicating gas: $4.5 - 3.0 = 1.5L$. Estimations of pneumothorax size may also be made from a CXR or CT chest.

9e) **What is the theoretical risk of flying, and how would she conventionally be advised?**

Oxygen saturation is normal; however, trapped gas within the thorax may put her at risk. Atmospheric pressure decreases with ascent to altitude (Fig. 9.5). At sea level atmospheric pressure is 101kPa (760mmHg).

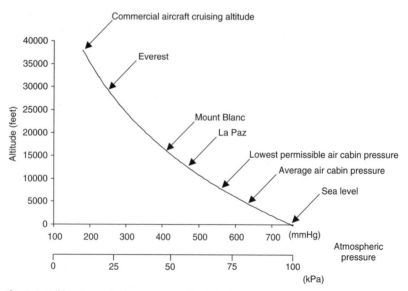

Fig. 9.6 Fall in atmospheric pressure with altitude.

Table 9.2 Screening for in-flight oxygen supplementation using SaO_2

Screening result	Recommendation
Sea level SaO_2 >95%	Oxygen not required
Sea level SaO_2 92–95% and no risk factor	Oxygen not required
Sea level SaO_2 92–95% and additional risk factor*	Perform hypoxic challenge test with arterial or capillary measurements of PaO_2
Sea level SaO_2 <92%	In-flight oxygen
Receiving supplemental oxygen at sea level	Increase the flow whilst in flight

* Additional risk factors are hypercapnia, FEV_1<50% predicted, lung cancer, fibrosis, scoliosis or respiratory muscle weakness, ventilator support, cerebrovascular or cardiac disease, within 6 weeks of discharge for an exacerbation of chronic lung or cardiac disease.

Commercial aircraft fly at about 30–40,000ft, but are required to pressurize the cabin to at least equivalent to 8000ft, or 73kPa (548mmHg). This is equivalent to breathing 15% oxygen at sea level. This drop in inspired oxygen tension is likely to be well-tolerated in this patient who is not hypoxic. In healthy people, arterial oxygen tension would be expected to fall to about 7.0–8.5kPa (53–64mmHg) with SaO_2 85–91%. Sea-level oxygen saturation is used as a screening test to determine whether supplementary oxygen is required in flight, according to British Thoracic Society recommendations (Table 9.2). If results are equivocal, a hypoxic challenge test breathing 15% inspired oxygen for 15 minutes may be carried out (Table 9.3). None of these recommendations are evidence-based.

Of much greater concern than hypoxia in this case is the expansion of trapped gas with increasing altitude. If allowed to expand freely, 1.5L of trapped gas in the pneumothoraces and cysts would increase inversely proportionately to the drop in atmospheric pressure, ie. to 1.5 × 760/548 = 2.1L. The theoretical risk is that increased air pressure inside the pneumothorax might lead to pain due to stripping of pleural adhesions, rupture and bleeding.

Table 9.3 Recommendation depending upon results of hypoxic challenge test (15% O_2 at sea level for 15 minutes)

Hypoxic challenge result	Recommendation
PaO_2 >7.4kPa (>55mmHg)	Oxygen not required
PaO_2 6.6–7.4kPa (50–55mmHg)	Borderline. A walk test may be helpful.
PaO_2 <6.6kPa	In-flight oxygen (2L/min)

Ordinarily the presence of a closed pneumothorax is an absolute contraindication to air flight, and arbitrarily patients are advised to wait 7 days after resolution of pneumothorax before air travel. In this case, however, the relative risk was considered low, since the pneumothorax was chronic, with pleural thickening and significant surrounding fibrosis reducing the risk of tissue tearing. Given the exceptional nature of this case, decompression in a hypobaric chamber was arranged, in step intervals to 10,000ft. Very minor chest discomfort was noted between 7500 and 8000ft, but she remained well. After discussion with the airline medical officer, she was permitted to fly, and had no adverse effects. In actual fact, cabin pressure is much more commonly pressurized to the equivalent of 3000 – 4000ft rather than the minimum of 8000ft.

Question

9f) Discuss issues to consider in her long-term management.

Answer

9f) **Discuss issues to consider in her long-term management.**

Patients with rare conditions such as LAM can often feel isolated, and may benefit from being put in touch with the relevant patient support group, LAM action (web address: www.lamaction.org).

Current treatments are aimed at managing complications:

- In the case of a second pneumothorax or a persistent air leak, early involvement of a thoracic surgeon is advised.

- Chylous collections tend to re-accumulate in a short time, if managed with simple drainage, and therefore obliteration of the pleural space or ligation of the thoracic duct is recommended. Reduction in lymphatic formation by strictly controlling dietary fat or substitution of fat by medium-chain triglycerides, which are absorbed from the intestine and carried in blood rather than lymphatics, is difficult for patients to adhere to and has generally not been very successful.

- Lung transplant may be considered in severe, end-stage LAM.

There are not yet treatments proven to slow disease progression. Oestrogen receptors are expressed aberrantly in the lungs, and so, theoretically, progesterone may slow progression, and oestrogen speed progression; however, hormonal treatments such as tamoxifen or medroxyprogesterone acetate have been found to be poorly effective, as have dietary manipulations. Pregnancy may put patients at risk due to hormonal effects, and because of the risk of respiratory compromise. Other approaches, such as use of the antiproliferative agent Rapamycin, are undergoing further evaluation.

Further reading

British Thoracic Society Standards of Care Committee (2002). Managing passengers with respiratory disease planning air travel: British Thoracic Society recommendations. *Thorax*; **57**: 289–304.

Glassberg MK (2004). Lymphangioleiomyomatosis. *Clinics in Chest Med*; **25**: 573–582.

Johnson S (2006). Lymphangioleiomyomatosis. Series 'rare interstitial lung diseases'. *Eur Respir*; **27**: 1056–1065.

'LAM action', patient support group and case registration web address: www.lamaction.org (accessed 1st September 2009)

Case 10

A 49-year-old man was referred from the haematology clinic with 18 months of breathlessness on exertion, a non-productive cough, and wheeze.

He had been diagnosed with follicular lymphoma 4 years previously, and had received extensive chemotherapy, as well as chest radiotherapy, a year later. One year after that, and 2 years prior to this presentation, he underwent an allogeneic bone marrow transplantation (BMT, sibling donor), which had been complicated by development of chronic graft-versus-host disease affecting his eyes and mouth. He had never smoked and there was no prior history of any lung disease.

His current medications included prednisolone 10mg once a day, cyclosporin 50mg twice a day, penicillin V 250mg twice a day, acyclovir 200mg twice a day, fluconazole 50mg once a day, co-trimoxazole 960mg 3 times a week, alendronic acid 70mg weekly, and omeprazole 20mg once a day. Becotide 200μg 2 puffs twice a day had been started by the referring team with little impact on his symptoms.

On examination his oxygen saturation was 97% on room air and he had scattered wheezes and squawks on auscultation.

Investigations

- FBC, U&Es and LFTs were all within normal limits
- CXR and pulmonary function tests are shown in Fig. 10.1 and Table 10.1.

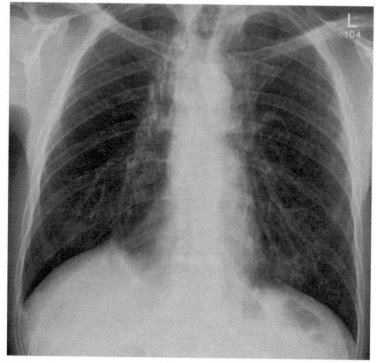

Fig. 10.1 CXR.

Table 10.1 Pulmonary function tests

	Measured	% Predicted
FEV$_1$(L)	2.4	65
FVC(L)	4.6	100
FEV$_1$/FVC ratio (%)	53	
VA(L)	5.4	77
TL$_{CO}$(mmol/min/kPa)	6.05	58
K$_{CO}$(mmol/min/kPa/L)	1.47	75

Questions

10a) What does (i) the CXR and (ii) the pulmonary function testing show?

10b) What is the likely diagnosis? What differential diagnoses would you consider?

10c) How would you manage this patient?

Answers

10a) **What does (i) the CXR and (ii) the pulmonary function testing show?**

The CXR shows hyper-inflation together with para-mediastinal fibrotic change in keeping with his previous radiotherapy exposure. Bi-apical pleural thickening and a tented right hemi-diaphragm are also present. (ii) His lung function tests show moderate airflow obstruction with reduced gas transfer.

10b) **What is the likely diagnosis? What differential diagnoses would you consider?**

The likely diagnosis is chronic pulmonary graft-versus-host-disease (GVHD) with bronchiolitis obliterans (also called obliterative bronchiolitis), mainly suggested by the obstructive defect and clinical context.

The differential diagnosis might include adult onset asthma or other causes of bronchiolitis. These are clearly less likely than chronic GVHD with pulmonary involvement, resulting in symptomatic airflow obstruction. The occurrence of bronchiolitis obliterans (BO) is not limited to those who develop chronic GVHD; it is also seen in some BMT patients without significant GVHD, and other lung insults, such as infection and irradiation, are thought to contribute. GVHD is usually associated with a severe form of BO which is very similar to that seen in lung transplant recipients.

The following points should be borne in mind:

◆ Minor asymptomatic decrements in lung function are common post-BMT, and a history of acute or chronic GVHD, older recipient age and early respiratory viral infection post-transplant are recognized risk factors.

◆ Symptomatic airflow obstruction post-BMT is more common in adults than children and occurs more frequently following allogeneic BMT. The exact pathogenesis remains elusive and disease is mild in most cases.

◆ Chronic (>100 days post-BMT) GVHD arises in up to 50% of patients who survive 6 months, and direct pulmonary involvement is common. The risk of other non-infectious pulmonary complications (see Table 10.2) is also increased by chronic GVHD, which itself is associated with marked immunosuppression, made worse by the drugs used to treat it. Clinically dyspnoea, a non-productive cough and wheeze (+/− crackles and squawks) are seen at a median post-transplant time of 5 months. The CXR may be normal, but lung function indicates airway obstruction unresponsive to bronchodilators. Histologically,

Table 10.2 Other pulmonary complications occurring late (>100 days) post-BMT

Infection	Risk is reduced with prophylaxis with antibiotics
Idiopathic pneumonia syndrome	Diagnosis of exclusion with associated high mortality
Diffuse alveolar haemorrhage	Underlying infection common, mortality high
Secondary alveolar proteinosis	Reported following transplantation for acute leukaemia. BAL positive for lipoproteins
Secondary malignancies	Underlying malignancy may relapse. Epstein-Barr virus related lymphoma can involve the lung
Radiation pneumonitis	Radiation induced pulmonary fibrosis, may take 6–24 months to develop and can develop in areas not irradiated
Pulmonary veno-occlusive disease	Rare. Patients dyspnoeic but lung function normal with no signs of infection. Right heart catheterization shows pulmonary hypertension and lung biopsy confirms the diagnosis

pulmonary GVHD may manifest as diffuse alveolar damage, lymphocytic interstitial pneumonia (LIP), lymphocytic bronchitis or bronchiolitis obliterans.

- Bronchiolitis obliterans may produce severe symptomatic airflow obstruction in between 2% and 14% of patients post-allogeneic BMT. Histologically the small airways are destroyed; fibromyxoid granulation tissue causes this small airway obliteration. It is almost exclusive to recipients with chronic GVHD, which has led to the hypothesis that the small airway obliteration is a pulmonary manifestation of GVHD (with bronchiolar epithelial cells targeted by cytotoxic donor T lymphocytes). The exact pathophysiology, however, is unknown; other factors postulated to mediate persistent small airway inflammation include viral infections, inadequate immunosuppression, low serum IgG, and gastro-oesophageal reflux.

10c) **How would you manage this patient?**

Management should include:

- Augmentation of immunosuppressive therapy (guided by the referring haematology team)
  - Increase in oral prednisolone dose (this is often tried first line)
  - Increase dose of other immunosuppressive agents

- Methotrexate, cyclosporin and azathioprine may be used in addition to prednisolone
- Thalidomide, methylprednisolone, hydroxychloroquine, tacrolimus and TNF antagonists have also been studied

♦ Optimization of bronchodilator medication
  - Long-acting bronchodilators
  - High-dose inhaled corticosteroids

♦ Exclusion of concomitant infection

♦ Prompt treatment of infection (to avoid decline in airflow obstruction and bronchiectatic exacerbations)

♦ High-resolution CT scan to confirm likely diagnosis and exclude alternatives

♦ Surveillance with monitoring of lung function/symptoms—the severity and progression of chronic GVHD related airflow obstruction is best assessed by regular monitoring of FEV_1.

There are no prospective studies to guide the definitive treatment of post-BMT airway obstruction. Most treatment approaches address underlying chronic GVHD with corticosteroids the mainstay of treatment for BO. Unfortunately BO is often poorly responsive to therapy.

Progress

Combination therapy (long-acting bronchodilators and inhaled corticosteroid) was commenced but, despite this, the FEV_1 fell from 2.4 to 1.9. A thoracic CT was performed (Fig. 10.2).

Questions

10d) What does the CT show?

10e) What would you do next?

10f) What other treatment strategies could be considered?

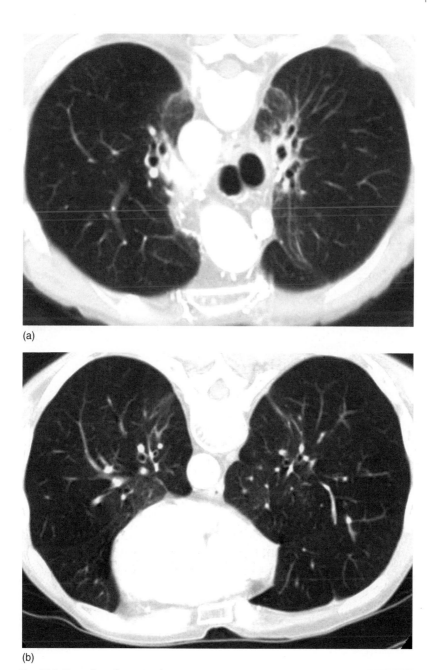

(a)

(b)

Fig. 10.2 Two slices from CT chest.

Answers

10d) **What does the CT show?**

His CT reveals para-mediastinal radiotherapy change with mild bron-chiectasis. A mosaic pattern of attenuation, consistent with areas of air-trapping, and subtle paucity of peripheral vascularity is seen.

10e) **What would you do next?**

The clinical and radiological picture is consistent with bronchiolitis obliterans and open lung biopsy for histological confirmation is not required. However, concomitant infection should be excluded as it is a common precipitant of symptomatic and spirometric deterioration (death due to severe chronic GVHD is usually a consequence of infectious complications).

Bronchoscopy with broncho-alveolar lavage (specimens sent for micro-scopy, culture for bacteria, mycobacteria and fungi, and cytology) should be performed next. Transbronchial biopsy for tissue histology is an option, but diagnostic sensitivity is limited as small airway involvement is often patchy.

10f) **What other treatment strategies could be considered?**

Other treatments to be considered include azithromycin. The anti-inflammatory action of macrolide antibiotics is well established, although the mechanism is poorly understood. Use of azithromycin has been shown to improve airflow limitation in patients with BO following BMT (although most evidence is available from patients with BO post-lung transplantation). The majority of responders will do so after three months of treatment. Hepatic impairment is a recognized complication of macrolides and liver function monitoring is advised.

Identification and treatment of gastro-oesophageal reflux, which may contribute to decline in lung function. Patients are at higher risk of reflux due to oesophageal involvement with GVHD and with the use of systemic corticosteroids.

All patients should receive annual influenza vaccination.

Progress

Pseudomonas species $<10^4$ organisms/ml were cultured from the BAL and a course of ciprofloxacin eradication therapy was completed. Azithromycin was started (250mg thrice weekly). Despite a period of stability, after 6 months his exercise tolerance fell (from 300 to 50 yards) and his FEV_1 dropped further. His prednisolone dose was increased to 30mg daily with little impact on his respiratory symptoms; ocular and mucosal symptoms remained under control.

Questions

10g) What would you do next?

10h) What is his prognosis?

Answers

10g) **What would you do next?**

- A therapeutic trial of higher dose azithromycin (250mg daily) can be considered
- Case reports of successful lung transplantation in selected patients with BO associated with chronic GVHD following allogeneic BMT, and refractory to conventional immunosuppressive therapy, have been published.

10h) **What is his prognosis?**

The prognosis of BO is poor, with an overall mortality of 65% at 3 years post-BMT. For patients with airflow obstruction *per se*, reported mortality rates of 9% at 3 years and 18% at 10 years; in those with chronic GVHD, rates of 22% at 3 years and 40% at 10 years have been noted (Chien *et al.* 2003).

Some patients with chronic pulmonary GVHD exhibit a fluctuating course with a remitting or relapsing pattern similar to other autoimmune diseases. A more progressive decline is usually seen in patients with BO with development of hypercapnic respiratory failure and death.

Early detection of airflow decline is important to allow prompt adjustment of immunomodulatory regimens and identification and treatment of exacerbating factors (e.g. infection and reflux) if present. Unfortunately, in spite of such focused approaches, the prognosis remains poor.

Further reading

Chien JW, Martin PJ, Gooley TA, Flowers ME, Heckbert SR, Nichols WG *et al.* (2003). Airflow obstruction after myeloablative allogeneic hematopoietic stem cell transplantation. *Am J Respir Crit* Care Med; **168**: 208–214.

Dudek AZ, Mahaseth H (2006). Hematopoietic stem cell transplant-related airflow obstruction. *Curr Opin Oncol*; **18**: 115–119.

Khalid M, Al Saghir A, Saleemi S, Al Dammas S, Zeitouni M, Al Mobeireek A *et al.* (2005). Azithromycin in bronchiolitis obliterans complicating bone marrow transplantation: a preliminary study. *Eur Respir J*; **25**: 490–493.

Case 11

A 53-year-old social worker was referred with a 2-year history of daily cough productive of small amounts of clear sputum. He had been given antibiotics every 3 months or so for episodes of increasing sputum purulence. He had no haemoptysis, exercise limitation or wheeze. Past history was of severe sinusitis in childhood requiring surgery, but he denied any childhood respiratory problems. At age 21 he had severe pneumonia and since then described colds 'going to his chest' in winter time but, until the last 2 years, had been well in-between these episodes. He was an ex-smoker of 10 years with a prior 25-pack year history. Systemic enquiry revealed no current upper airway or GI symptoms (e.g. bloating, fatty stools or difficulty maintaining weight) but he had intermittent arthralgia affecting his wrists, elbows and shoulders. He had 2 children and denied any family history of respiratory disease. On examination he weighed 91.7kg, BMI 29, there were some course crackles in the right base, but otherwise was completely normal.

Investigations

- Hb 13.8g/dL, WCC 9.33×10^9/L, platelets 404×10^9/L
- ESR 22mm/h, CRP 6mg/L, U&E, glucose, LFT normal
- Sputum culture, no growth
- Pulmonary function (Table 11.1).

Table 11.1 Pulmonary function tests

	Measured	% Predicted
FEV$_1$(L)	2.7	73
FVC(L)	4.8	102
FEV$_1$/FVC(%)	53	
FRC(L)	5.5	151
RV(L)	3.9	171
TLC(L)	9.0	123
VA(L)	5.9	81
TL$_{CO}$(mmol/min/kPa)	9.44	90
K$_{CO}$(mmol/min/kPa/L)	1.6	112

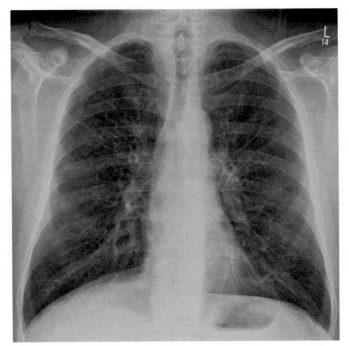

Fig. 11.1 CXR.

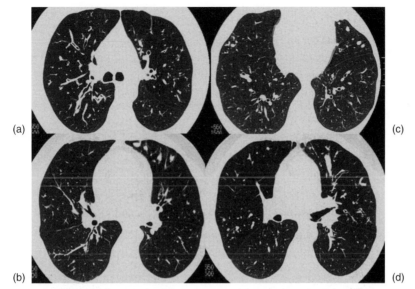

(a)

(b)

(c)

(d)

Fig. 11.2 Four slices from HRCT thorax.

Questions

11a) Interpret the lung function tests.

11b) Interpret the CXR.

11c) Interpret the HRCT images.

11d) What is the differential diagnosis?

11e) What key part of the history has to be clarified to aid a clinical diagnosis?

11f) What further investigations are needed?

Answers

11a) **Interpret the lung function tests.**

The lung function (Table 11.1) shows airflow obstruction, and static lung volumes show hyperinflation and air trapping. Reversibility testing has not been performed.

11b) **Interpret the CXR.**

The CXR shows mildly hyperinflated lung fields. There is bronchial wall thickening throughout both lung fields.

11c) **Interpret the HRCT images.**

The HRCT slices (Fig. 11.2) show features of generalized bronchiectasis, with dilated airways, bronchial wall thickening and mucous plugging.

11d) **What is the differential diagnosis?**

Differential diagnosis includes the causes of generalized bronchiectasis:

- Immune deficiency—primary (e.g. hypogammaglobulinaemia, common variable immunodeficiency) or secondary (HIV, CLL)
- Post-infective (whooping cough, TB, severe pneumonia; although these often produce more patchy, or localized, bronchiectasis)
- Mucociliary clearance abnormalities
- Primary ciliary dyskinesia
- Young's syndrome
- Cystic fibrosis
- Connective tissue disease (RA, SLE, Sjögren's syndrome)
- Inflammatory bowel disease
- Yellow nail syndrome
- Idiopathic.

11e) **What key part of the history has to be clarified to aid a clinical diagnosis?**

The family history must be clarified. Males with CF are infertile, but the patient has 2 children. On revisiting this issue it transpired that the patient's children had been adopted because he was infertile. Furthermore, his younger sister had died at the age of 5 with an unknown, undiagnosed illness associated with severe pneumonia and malabsorption. His mother died from breast cancer in her 50s and his father died aged 62 following an MI. This makes cystic fibrosis a likely cause for his bronchiectasis.

11f) **What further investigations are needed?**

With knowledge of the full family history, investigations can be targeted at confirming the diagnosis of CF. Other investigations, looking for other underlying causes of generalized bronchiectasis (such as immunoglobulins, auto-antibody screen), are not essential at present. CF must be considered in all adults presenting with otherwise unexplained generalized bronchiectasis.

The most appropriate initial investigation would be genotyping for the common CF mutations. Over 1000 different mutations in the cystic fibrosis transmembrane conductance regulator (CFTR) gene are recognized to cause clinical disease, with homozygosity for ΔF508 mutation the most common (approximately 67%).

Genotyping revealed our patient to be a compound heterozygote for ΔF508 and R117H. The clinical spectrum for this mutation is highly variable but usually mild, with some adult patients asymptomatic (detected by screening following a sibling diagnosis of CF). Other presentations include mild cough, through to clinical bronchiectasis as demonstrated here, to rarely more severe fatal disease. Returning to our patient's family history, this raises intriguing questions about his sister's genotype. ΔF508 homozygosity invariably causes malabsorption, whereas the R117H and most other mutations permit partial CFTR function and are only rarely associated with pancreatic insufficiency. If she had the same genotype as our patient, her malabsorption would not have been due to CF. For this she would have had to be homozygous for ΔF508 and therefore one of her parents would have to have been a compound heterozygote ΔF508/R117 (and apparently asymptomatic) and the other a simple carrier of the ΔF508 mutation (frequency in the general population 1/25). Alternatively, our patient's sister could have died of other causes.

In the clinical context of our patient, if genotyping studies for common mutations had been negative, other supporting evidence for a clinical diagnosis of CF would be sought. Here a sweat test could be helpful, but results in adults are more likely to be borderline, as the reference ranges for normal sweat concentrations are wider and higher. A repeatedly positive test would, however, be diagnostic (chloride sweat concentration of >60 mmol/L). Some CF mutations associated with milder disease may produce a near normal, or even normal, sweat test. False-negatives are thus possible (although less common than false-positives) and the test should be repeated in a patient with a phenotype suggestive of CF.

He has the clinical triad of Young's syndrome (bronchiectasis, sinusitis and infertility). Separating this from CF requires normal sweat chloride level and pancreatic function; and from primary ciliary dyskinesia (PCD) by normal ciliary ultrastructure. The cause of Young's syndrome is unknown, but the respiratory secretions are excessively viscid leading to prolonged mucociliary transport.

Another diagnosis to consider in this context, had the genotype been negative, would be primary ciliary dyskinesia (PCD) which is characterized by bronchiectasis, chronic sinusitis and middle ear disease (although patients are not invariably infertile). When PCD is associated with dextro-cardia (50% of cases) it assumes the eponym Kartagener's syndrome. Ciliary function can be assessed by light microscopy (beat frequency) and electron microscopy (ultrastructure) of a nasal brush biopsy (only available in specialist centres). An alternative is to perform a saccharin test, where a small (0.5mm) particle from a saccharin tablet is placed 1cm behind, or under, the front edge of the inferior turbinate. The patient sits quietly, should not sniff, looks down and reports when sweetness is tasted. Beyond 30 minutes is considered abnormal.

Further reading

Massie RJ, Poplawski N, Wilcken B, Goldblatt J, Byrnes C, Robertson C (2001). Intron-8 polythymidine sequence in Australasian individuals with CF mutations R117H and R117C. *ERJ*; **17**: 1195–2000.

Wilson R (2003). Bronchiectasis. In: Gibson GJ, Geddes DM, Costabel U *et al.* (eds) *Respiratory Medicine* (3rd edn). Saunders, London, chapter 49, pp. 1445–1464.

Hodson M, Geddes D, Bush A (eds) (2007). *Cystic Fibrosis* (3rd edn). Hodder Arnold, London.

Case 12

A 53-year-old lady presented to her GP with a lower respiratory tract infection following a holiday in Spain. Two courses of antibiotics produced little response. Because she was wheezing, and had a history of exercise wheeze in the past, she received beclomethasone and salbutamol inhalers; in addition, her atenolol for hypertension was stopped. This produced a short-lived improvement but wheezing and intermittent dizziness continued, despite various changes in asthma therapy. Finally, despite a normal peak flow, she received a course of oral steroids pending referral to the clinic.

In clinic she brought a peak flow chart showing values varying between 400 and 500 L/m, but with no hint of morning dipping. She had never smoked, had a past history of sinus problems, had no children (but several miscarriages) and was divorced. She slept well. Recent routine haematology and biochemistry (including thyroid function) were normal.

On examination

She appeared anxious and was tachypnoeic at rest. Resting arterial SaO_2 was 99%. Examination was otherwise normal. She was exercised by stepping up and down a 9in block; she immediately became breathless, managing only 8 steps, and her breathing was irregular throughout. Her SaO_2 remained at 99% during and after the exercise. Doing spirometry made her dizzy, Table 12.1.

Table 12.1 Pulmonary function tests

	Measured	% Predicted
FEV_1	2.9(l)	110%
FVC	3.2(l)	108%

Investigations
CXR and ECG normal.

Questions

12a) What is the most likely diagnosis?

12b) What test would be appropriate next?

Answers

12a) **What is the most likely diagnosis?**

Given the normal lung function and normoxia, the degree of dyspnoea was out of proportion, particularly on mild exercise, when the dyspnoea became acutely worse before any significant energy expenditure. The supra-normal SaO_2 (>98%) is perhaps of interest too. This raises the possibility of psychogenic dyspnoea (dysfunctional breathing, or hyper-ventilation syndrome, all these terms are used interchangeably). This is both a diagnosis of exclusion, as well as requiring the presence of a likely explanation for this psychological response.

12b) **What test would be appropriate next?**

As a diagnostic test, some recommend asking the patient to deliberately hyperventilate to see if they develop the same symptoms, such as dizzi-ness, numbness and tingling of the lips and extremities, and a sense of impending doom. This does not always work. Arterial blood gases at rest can be very useful. They showed the following:

- pH, 7.48
- $PaCO_2$ (kPa), 3.62
- PaO_2 (kPa), 15.1
- $[HCO_3]^-$ (mmol/L), 21.7
- Base excess (mmol/L), −3.3.

Questions

12c) What do the blood gases tell you about the degree of over (or under) ventilation, and for how long it might have been going on?

12d) What is this patient's alveolar to arterial gradient for oxygen?

12e) Do these blood gas results support the diagnosis of hyperventilation syndrome?

12f) What theories are there as to the cause of this syndrome?

12g) What are the important alternative diagnoses to exclude, and why do they not seem likely in this lady?

12h) What approaches are available to manage this syndrome?

Answers

12c) **What do the blood gases tell you about the degree of over (or under) ventilation, and for how long it might have been going on?**

The $PaCO_2$ is low, and therefore there is alveolar hyperventilation; there is not a low PaO_2 (in fact slightly high), so that hypoxia is not the cause of the hyperventilation. There is a small base deficit suggesting a renal metabolic compensation for the respiratory alkalosis, indicating some chronicity to the hyperventilation.

12d) **What is this patient's alveolar to arterial gradient for oxygen?**

The alveolar to arterial gradient is normal at 0.4kPa. In young people up to 2kPa is considered normal, and up to 3kPa in the elderly.

The alveolar to arterial gradient for oxygen is essentially how much the arterial PaO_2 is less than it ought to be, given the alveolar PO_2, which is predicted from the $PaCO_2$ (i.e. the more you ventilate, the lower the $PaCO_2$ and the higher the PaO_2 ought to be). Therefore, it is calculated by first correcting the $PaCO_2$ for the respiratory quotient (CO_2 produced, divided by oxygen consumed, usually 0.8), subtract it from the inspired oxygen pressure (less water vapour pressure, about 1kPa) and then subtract the actual PaO_2 from it. Thus in this case:

A−a gradient = (20−3.62/0.8)−15.1 = 0.4kPa.

12e) **Do these blood gas results support the diagnosis of hyperventilation syndrome?**

This indicates there are no low V/Q units, indicating neither areas of lung with relative underventilation compared to perfusion, nor right-to-left shunting. This, together with the low $PaCO_2$, strongly supports hyperventilation with no intrinsic lung abnormality.

12f) **What theories are there as to the cause of this syndrome?**

The explanations for hyperventilation syndrome are varied. It appears to be one of several symptom complexes reflecting anxiety and panic attacks, sometimes called somatization. These include diarrhoea and abdominal pain, episodes of sharp chest pain, palpitations, sweating, headaches and so on. A significant proportion of patients with agoraphobia have hyperventilation syndrome. Once established, fears of serious underlying disease seem to maintain it. In the respiratory version, some preceding respiratory event, such as a chest infection, or episode of asthma, generates breathlessness and anxiety which persists after the original problem has resolved.

The hyperventilation and consequent alkalosis generate a variety of symptoms that concern the patient (dizziness from the cerebral vasoconstriction, general tiredness and weakness, numbness and tingling, dyspnoea), which produce more hyperventilation and more anxiety. The hypocapnia is said to sometimes cause wheeziness. Functional laryngeal dysfunction can occur, with inspiratory stridor. Occasionally the episodes may be self-terminated by loss of consciousness from the hypocapnia-induced cerebral vasoconstriction. It can exist in an episodic form, or more chronically when dyspnoea occurs most of the time, and a base deficit develops. This case is more at the chronic end of the spectrum. It is more common in women, and usually occurs between the ages of 15 and 55. This patient had a history of respiratory symptoms and a more recent acute event. She had no demonstrable objective abnormalities (apart from persistently high SaO_2), a bizarre breathing pattern, and no exercise desaturation.

12g) **What are the important alternative diagnoses to exclude, and why do they not seem likely in this lady?**

It is important not to miss other diagnoses that present with few clues (and no fall in SaO_2 on exercise to the point of breathlessness) when making a diagnosis of hyperventilation syndrome, e.g.

+ Very mild asthma
+ Thyrotoxicosis
+ Primary pulmonary hypertension
+ Early interstitial lung disease with a normal CXR
+ Early heart failure
+ Pulmonary emboli.

The last four, however, would normally be expected to produce a fall in SaO_2 following sufficient exercise to provoke breathlessness.

Thus an HRCT might be indicated, but unnecessary investigations will increase the patient's view that 'the doctors think something is wrong'.

Calcium levels should be checked, as hypocalcaemia may cause similar symptoms to alkalosis: weakness, carpopedal spasm, and parasthesiae.

Early interstitial lung disease is unlikely here, given the supranormal spirometry; asthma seems unlikely given the normal FEV_1/VC ratio and unconvincing peak flow chart. Primary pulmonary hypertension seems unlikely given the normal ECG and no exercise hypoxia. Heart failure seems unlikely with normal sleep and an uncharacteristic

Table 12.1 Nijmegen score. A score over 22 is highly suggestive of hyperventilation syndrome

Before treatment	Never 0	Rarely 1	Some-times 2	Often 3	Very often 4
Chest pain			✓		
Feeling tense				✓	
Blurred vision		✓			
Dizzy spells			✓		
Feeling confused			✓		
Faster/deeper breathing					✓
Shortness of breath				✓	
Tight feeling in the chest					✓
Bloated feeling in the stomach			✓		
Tingling fingers	✓				
Unable to breath deeply				✓	
Stiff fingers or arms			✓		
Tight feeling around mouth	✓				
Cold hands or feet	✓				
Heart racing (palpitations)				✓	
Feeling anxious				✓	
Total score = 34					
After treatment	**Never 0**	**Rarely 1**	**Some-times 2**	**Often 3**	**Very often 4**
Chest pain	✓				
Feeling tense		✓			
Blurred vision	✓				
Dizzy spells	✓				
Feeling confused	✓				
Faster/deeper breathing	✓				
Shortness of breath			✓		
Tight feeling in the chest		✓			
Bloated feeling in the stomach	✓				
Tingling fingers	✓				
Unable to breath deeply	✓				
Stiff fingers or arms	✓				
Tight feeling around mouth	✓				
Cold hands or feet	✓				
Heart racing (palpitations)	✓				
Feeling anxious	✓				
Total score = 4					

pattern of dyspnoea. The immediate dyspnoea on attempting exercise, and the irregular pattern during it, suggest a psychogenic origin.

12h) **What approaches are available to manage this syndrome?**

Treatment can be difficult with great resistance to accepting that there is nothing physically wrong, and accepting that not reacting to stress with hyperventilation will help. Sometimes, firm reassurance that nothing is structurally amiss, and a careful explanation as to how hyperventilation syndrome comes about, will work. The explanation needs to acknowledge that there is a problem, which is not 'all in the mind', and that it has arisen from real pathology, which has resolved, but that the body is now reacting inappropriately. More formally, this could be delivered as cognitive behaviour therapy.

Some will use a short course of sedatives to demonstrate to the patient that it can be stopped, which may help convince the patient of its origins.

Physiotherapists have developed useful approaches to helping patients focus their anxiety away from their breathing. Examples include: breathing slowly through the nose, using the diaphragm rather than the upper chest; avoiding sighing and yawning; trying specific relaxation techniques; and placing the hands over the cheeks during attacks (the cold clammy hands are thought to inhibit inspiration via the diving reflex—stimulation of the trigeminal area with cold).

The Nijmegen score (Table 12.1) can be useful to follow patients, assess their responses to treatment and as a patient education tool. This patient was treated by a physiotherapist skilled in this area, and the patient's score sheets, before and after treatment, are shown in Table 12.1.

Further reading

www.physiohypervent.org (accessed 1st September 2009)

Case 13

A 31-year-old man presented to the emergency department with dyspnoea, slowly progressive over a period of 3 months, associated with fatigue, anorexia and 2-stone weight loss. One week before presentation he developed night sweats. He was otherwise fit and well, with no relevant past medical or family history. He was Indian and had moved to the UK 5 years previously. On examination he was febrile, tachypnoeic (20/min) with oxygen saturations of 96% on room air, and signs of a large left pleural effusion. A BCG scar was present in the right deltoid area.

Investigations

- Mild leukocytosis
- Raised inflammatory markers (CRP = 98mg/L, ESR = 66mm/h)
- CXR, Fig. 13.1.

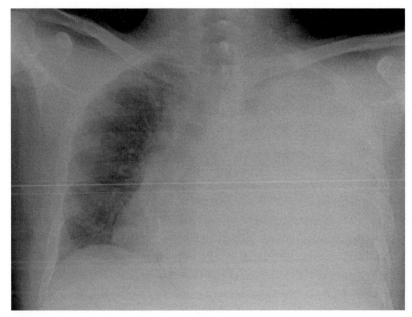

Fig. 13.1 CXR.

Questions

13a) Provide a differential diagnosis for this presentation.

13b) What is the most appropriate next diagnostic step?

Answers

13a) **Provide a differential diagnosis for this presentation.**
Differential diagnosis of massive effusion. Although heart failure may present with unilateral effusion, it is unlikely to cause an effusion of this size. The main differentials to consider are, therefore:

- TB pleuritis—in an Indian presenting with progressive symptoms, large effusion and systemic illness, this is the most likely diagnosis. TB pleuritis is usually associated with small to moderate sized collections but large effusions may occur. TB pleuritis is the result of an immunological reaction in the pleural space to mycobacteria, and should not be confused with TB empyema

- Malignancy—around 70% of massive (>2/3 hemithorax) effusions are due to primary or secondary malignancy. Tissue types to be considered in this age group include lymphoma, germ cell tumours and testicular cancer. A systemic inflammatory reaction is not uncommon

- Parapneumonic effusion/empyema—the prolonged (3-month) history of symptoms does not rule out pleural infection (especially with anaerobic organisms), which may run an indolent course. Such a massive effusion is against the diagnosis of frank empyema (the patient would be likely to be much more unwell).

- Acute trauma and haemothorax may cause a massive effusion, but the history is too prolonged.

13b) **What is the most appropriate next diagnostic step?**
Diagnostic pleural aspiration is the next step to narrow the differential. With a large effusion, the initial attempt can be made 'blind'. If pleural fluid is not obtained at the first attempt (by an experienced operator), image guidance is required.

Progress

Diagnostic pleural aspiration was undertaken.

Investigations

- Appearance: straw-coloured, no odour
- Biochemistry:
  - pH 7.43
  - Glucose 3.3mmol/L

- Protein 53g/L
- LDH 431IU/L (serum normal 13–250)
- Cytology:
  - Benign reactive mesothelial cells
  - Few mature lymphocytes
  - No malignant cells seen
- Microbiology:
  - Gram stain negative
  - ZN stain negative.

Questions

13c) Comment on the pleural fluid biochemical parameters.

13d) Comment on the pleural fluid microbiology and cytology results in terms of differential diagnosis.

13e) What is the next stage in diagnosis / management?

Answers

13c) **Comment on the pleural fluid biochemical parameters.**

Pleural fluid biochemistry:

- ◆ Exudate on the basis of Light's criteria (see case 22) (assuming serum protein and LDH to be normal). In this situation this does not aid in narrowing the differential diagnosis, as the main differentials are exudates.
- ◆ Suggestive of an inflammatory exudate (high LDH indicative of high cell turnover).
- ◆ Normal pH and glucose are strong indicators that this is not due to bacterial pleural infection.
- ◆ Pleural fluid pH of <7.2 and a glucose of around 1mmol/L are usual for complicated parapneumonic effusion or empyema (also seen in some cases of malignancy, oesophageal perforation, rheumatoid disease and systemic lupus erythematosis).
- ◆ Glucose level of 3.3mmol/L (low-normal) would be typical of TB pleuritis.

13d) **Comment on the pleural fluid microbiology and cytology results in terms of differential diagnosis.**

Pleural fluid microbiology and cytology:

- ◆ Negative Gram and ZN stains do not rule out bacterial or mycobacterial infection, as effusions may be mainly reactive to the presence of a few bacteria.
- ◆ Up to 40% of empyemas are Gram and culture negative.
- ◆ Only the minority of TB effusions are ZN positive.
- ◆ Absence of malignant cells does not rule out malignancy (40% cytology negative on first aspiration).
- ◆ TB pleuritis typically associated with a lymphocyte predominant cell population; up to 10% of cases are polymorph predominant.

13e) **What is the next stage in diagnosis / management?**

Management:

- ◆ The diagnosis is not established and there is no gross respiratory embarrassment, therefore complete drainage of pleural fluid (as was done here) is unnecessary and makes subsequent pleural biopsy hazardous.
- ◆ There are no biochemical parameters (pH <7.2, glucose <2mmol/L) indicating pleural infection requiring drainage.

- Draining a limited amount of pleural fluid for patient comfort would be reasonable.
- Pleural biopsy (non-image guided, e.g. Abram's, image guided or thoracoscopic) or contrast enhanced thoracic CT (to highlight the pleural surfaces) would be the next step.
- Given the high likelihood of TB pleuritis, closed (e.g. Abram's) pleural biopsy would be reasonable (overall sensitivity of ZN stain or culture and histology of ~80%), although trial evidence suggests that thoracoscopy has a far higher sensitivity (approaching 100%).

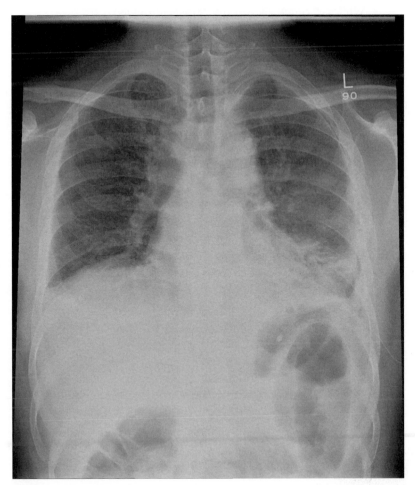

Fig. 13.2 CXR post drainage.

Progress

The patient was started on broad-spectrum antibiotics, a chest drain was inserted and the effusion freely drained for presumed pleural infection. Twenty-four hours after drain insertion, a CXR was performed (Fig. 13.2).

Five days later the patient was afebrile and clinically improved. Blood cultures and pleural fluid cultures were negative and he was discharged home with out-patient follow-up in 4 weeks.

One week after discharge, he was admitted to the respiratory unit with an acute illness characterized by high fevers, sweats and malaise.

Investigations

- ◆ White cell count, 28×10^6/ml, 90% neutrophils
- ◆ Raised inflammatory markers (CRP >160mg/L, ESR, 13mm/h)

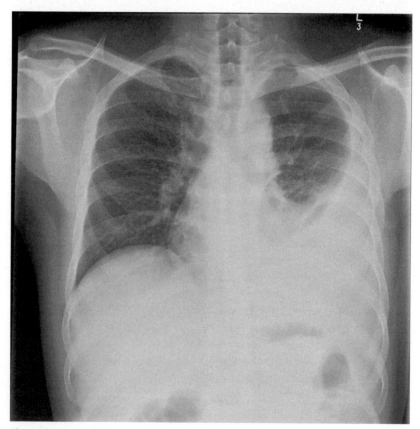

Fig. 13.3 Repeat CXR.

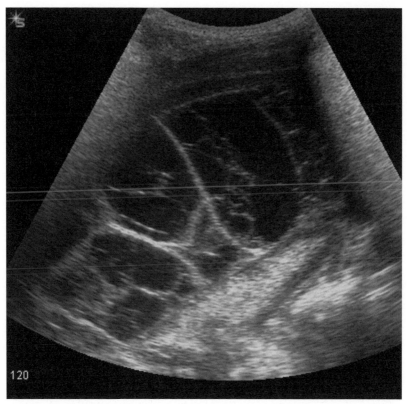

Fig. 13.4 Septated collection.

- Pleural fluid parameters at this stage:
  - Appearance, turbid
  - Biochemistry, pH 6.9
  - Glucose, 1.0mmol/L
  - Protein, 50g/L LDH 5467IU/L
- Thoracic ultrasound: see Fig. 13.4.

Questions

13f) Comment on the post drainage CXR (Fig. 13.2).

13g) What is the most likely diagnosis for this second presentation?

13h) Give the most important immediate steps in management.

Answers

13f) **Comment on the post drainage CXR (Fig. 13.2).**

Shows a chest drain *in situ* in the left lower zone, some left basal consolidation and pleural reaction, and a bulky left hilar/aorto-pulmonary window area suggestive of lymphadenopathy.

13g) **What is the most likely diagnosis for this second presentation?**

The most likely diagnosis for this second presentation is pleural infection (possibly iatrogenic given the previous chest drain), consistent with the:

- Pleural fluid biochemistry (suggestive of complicated para-pneumonic effusion)
- Appearance (turbidity suggestive of above)
- Radiology (septations on ultrasound).

13h) **Give the most important immediate steps in management.**

Management of pleural infection:

- Broad-spectrum antibiotics to cover likely pathogens, i.e. Gram-positive, Gram-negative and anaerobic bacteria, including cover in this situation for possible MRSA
- Same-day chest drainage (image guided, if necessary)
- TB pleuritis was not excluded on the previous admission, therefore obtaining pleural tissue should now be considered.

Progress

Broad-spectrum antibiotics were instituted, closed pleural biopsies performed and a chest drain inserted.

Investigations (48h later)

- Pleural fluid microbiology—profuse growth of coagulase-negative *Staphylococcus*, sensitive to flucloxacillin
- Closed pleural biopsies—necrotizing granulomatous inflammation but microbiologically negative (Fig. 13.5).

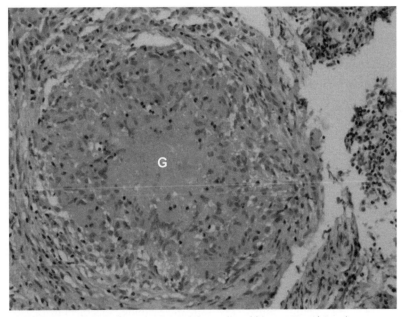

Fig. 13.5 One TB caseating granuloma (G) on pleural biopsy, H and E stain.

Questions

13i) What is now your diagnosis?

13j) What antibiotics should this patient now be given?

13k) Comment on the negative microbiology in terms of whether treatment for TB should be considered.

Answers

13i) **What is now your diagnosis?**

Diagnosis:

- ◆ Definite acute bacterial pleural infection (staphylococcal)
- ◆ In association with TB pleuritis.

13j) **What antibiotics should this patient now be given?**

Antibiotics:

- ◆ Pleural infection is often associated with mixed bacterial pathogens
- ◆ Broad-spectrum antibiotics to cover likely pathogens, i.e. Gram-positive, Gram-negative, anaerobes, cover in this situation for possible MRSA.

13k) **Comment on the negative microbiology in terms of whether treatment for TB should be considered.**

TB pleuritis:

- ◆ Closed pleural biopsy (ZN stain and histology together) has a diagnostic sensitivity of around 60% for TB pleuritis
- ◆ If microbiological culture is added (waiting 6–8 weeks) this increases to around 80%
- ◆ Anti-tuberculosis therapy should be started on the basis of the clinical history and the histology result, in the absence of positive microbiology.

Progress

Satisfactory fluid drainage was achieved. After 5 days of intravenous antibiotic therapy he was commenced on quadruple anti-tuberculosis chemotherapy, tolerating this well. He was discharged home with an appointment in the out-patient clinic in 2 weeks to assess response.

Ten days later he was re-admitted with progressive dyspnoea. A CXR showed a residual left-sided pleural effusion. A thoracic CT scan was performed (Fig. 13.6).

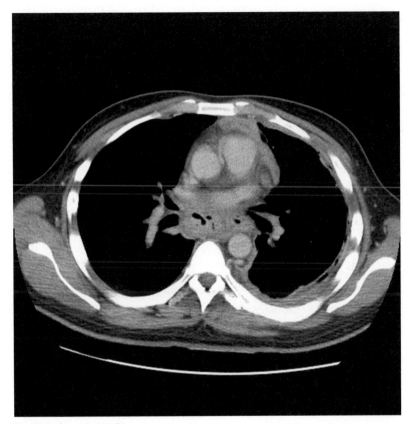

Fig. 13.6 Thoracic CT slice.

Questions

13l) What are the abnormalities on the thoracic CT scan (Fig. 13.6)?

13m) What two diagnostic tests could be performed at this stage to confirm the diagnosis?

Answers

13l) **What are the abnormalities on the thoracic CT scan (Fig. 13.6)?**

Thoracic CT (Fig. 13.7):

- ◆ Enhancing left pleural effusion
- ◆ Two separate, non-dependant areas of gas within it, suggestive of a loculated pleural space
- ◆ There is free air present in the mediastinum
- ◆ This combination is suggestive of oesophageal perforation and infected pleural effusion

13m) **What two diagnostic tests could be performed at this stage to confirm the diagnosis?**

Diagnostic tests:

- ◆ Pleural fluid amylase:
  - • Raised pleural fluid amylase (i.e. greater than serum normal range) confirms the diagnosis of oesophageal perforation, caused by saliva entering the pleural space through the perforation
  - • Raised pleural fluid amylase levels may also be seen in acute pancreatitis and malignancy (adenocarcinoma)

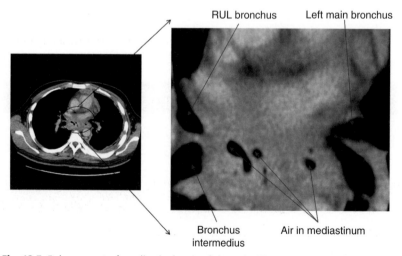

RUL bronchus   Left main bronchus

Bronchus   Air in mediastinum
intermedius

Fig. 13.7 Enlargement of mediastinal area of thoracic CT.

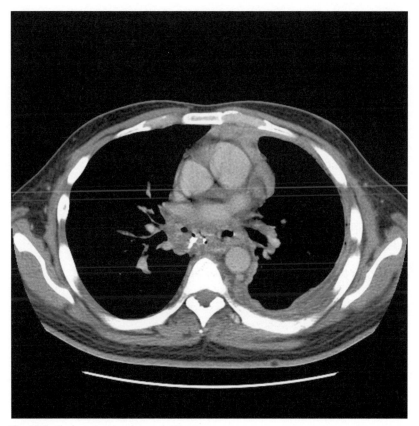

Fig. 13.8 Oral contrast-enhanced CT scan.

- Oesophageal perforation can be distinguished by conducting isoenzyme analysis of the pleural fluid, revealing amylase of salivary origin
- Oral contrast-enhanced thoracic CT reveals contrast in the mediastinum (and perhaps pleural fluid) confirming the diagnosis (Fig. 13.8).

Questions

13n) What is the differential diagnosis of this condition?

13o) How would you manage this patient?

Answers

13n) **What is the differential diagnosis of this condition?**

Causes of oesophageal perforation:

+ Malignant oesophageal perforation
+ Iatrogenic (post-OGD, post-oesophageal dilatation)
+ Post-upper GI surgery
+ Oesophageal rupture (Boerhaave's syndrome)
+ Malignant/necrotic mediastinal node compression.

13o) **How would you manage this patient?**

Management of oesophageal rupture:

+ Surgical referral for possible repair
+ Upper GI rest (feeding jejunostomy or TPN)
+ Treat infection (mediastinitis, pleural infection).

Progress

+ Referred for upper GI surgical opinion
+ Endoscopy—3 × 3cm hole in the distal oesophagus, adjacent to large volume mediastinal necrotic node disease on CT
+ Laparotomy: omental biopsies revealed caseating granuloma and a feeding jejunostomy was inserted
+ Nil by mouth (6 weeks), broad-spectrum antibiotics (4 weeks) and TB quadruple therapy (6-month regime)
+ Chest drain remained *in situ* for 2 weeks, no further pleural fluid accumulation
+ Discharged at 6 weeks on a normal diet and completed TB therapy without complication
+ Now fully recovered and working again.

Final diagnosis

TB pleuritis, subsequent iatrogenic empyema and subsequent oesophageal perforation secondary to necrotic TB mediastinal lymph nodes.

Case 14

A 78-year-old man was referred for continuous positive airway pressure (CPAP) therapy. He had developed snoring and witnessed apnoeas over the past 5 years (having had an unsuccessful uvulopalatopharyngoplasty), along with excessive daytime sleepiness over the last year (Epworth Sleepiness Score, 16/24). He had lost 5kg (BMI of 21). Three years previously he had an ineffective prostatectomy for urinary retention and dribbling. He had started shouting during sleep and thrashing around in bed. His wife thought that he had 'slowed up' over the last year. He was now finding it difficult to play the piano, but put this down to his being 78. On more direct questioning he described dizziness on getting out of bed in the mornings, after meals and if he got out of a chair too quickly. He had been impotent for several years and noticed he no longer sweated. He was taking no medications.

A sleep study was performed recording oxygen saturation, pulse rate, sound levels (Fig. 14.1) along with a video-recording available for reviewing, if necessary.

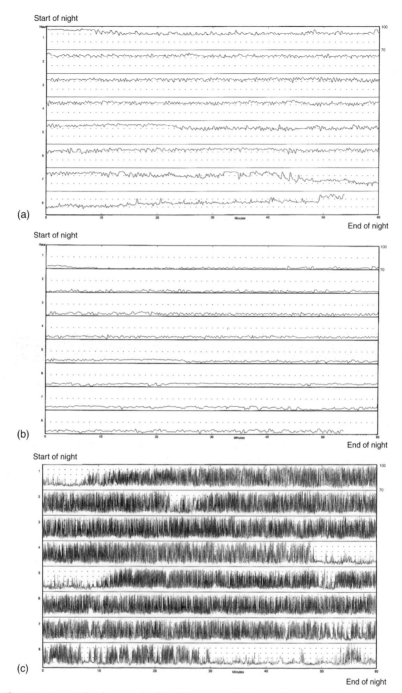

Fig. 14.1 Overnight sleep study. (a) Eight sequential hours of overnight oximetry (each scale 70–100% SaO$_2$), starting top-left and ending bottom-right. (b) Eight sequential hours of overnight pulse rate (each scale 50–170BPM), starting top-left and ending bottom-right. (c) Eight sequential hours of overnight snoring (each scale 30–80dB), starting top-left and ending bottom-right.

Analysis

- ◆ Oximetry:
  - • Mean level, 91.1 %
  - • >4% SaO_2 dips/h, 13.1
  - • Lowest SaO_2, 77 %
- ◆ Pulse:
  - • Mean level, 66BPM
  - • Standard deviation, 4.1BPM
- ◆ Sound:
  - • Time>70dB, 361min.

Questions

14a) Do the tracings (Fig. 14.1) show obstructive sleep apnoea/hypopnoea, if so, how severe is it?

14b) Why is the heart rate tracing unusual for obstructive sleep apnoea?

14c) What is the diagnosis and why, what further information would have been available from listening to the video?

Answers

14a) **Do the tracings (Fig. 14.1) show obstructive sleep apnoea/hypopnoea, if so, how severe is it?**

The oximetry tracing shows oscillating SaO_2, which could be due to a variety of causes, both central and obstructive. On this tracing alone further differentiation is not possible with any confidence. The noise tracing (once verified as snoring) would of course strongly support obstructive sleep apnoea/hypopnoea, and this could be further verified by watching and listening to a segment of the video. The fact that he is not obese reduces the probability of conventional OSA. The severity is considerable as it extends throughout most of the night; however, because the size of the dips often does not reach the >4% threshold to be counted, the oxygen desaturation index (ODI) is only 13.1/h and markedly understates the severity of the sleep apnoea. This usually occurs when a patient with OSA is thin.

The rate at which the SaO_2 falls during an apnoea depends on lung stores of oxygen and the rate at which oxygen is consumed—in thin people, the FRC is proportionately larger than in obese individuals, and their metabolic rate is proportionately lower. This means that in the more obese, the SaO_2 falls faster during an apnoea and vice versa. Thus a negative screening sleep study, particularly if relying on computer derived indices, rather than looking at the tracing, will be more likely to be *falsely negative* in thinner individuals. In contrast, *false positive* screening oximetry tracings are more likely if someone is obese, and/or the starting SaO_2 baseline is low (<93%, e.g. at altitude or with COPD), as it is easier to drop the SaO_2 by 4% with more minor oscillations in ventilation if you are already on the steep part of the haemoglobin dissociation curve.

14b) **Why is the heart rate tracing unusual for obstructive sleep apnoea?**

Normally the heart rate rises with every arousal following an apnoeic/hypopnoeic event. This is because the obstructive event is terminated by activation of the brainstem by the arousal stimuli, which increases pharyngeal muscle tone and simultaneously activates the autonomic centres. Usually the arousal then spreads through the cortex, to a varying degree, producing the sleep fragmentation. On inspection, his heart-rate tracing shows very little oscillation (as also evidenced by the very low standard deviation, <10%). Often this is due to the patient taking β blockers, which was not the case here.

14c) **What is the diagnosis and why, what further information would have been available from listening to the video?**

The diagnosis is Shy–Drager syndrome (or multi-system atrophy); the sound tracing of the sleep study must be listened to in order to identify laryngeal obstruction (stridulous), as opposed to the more common pharyngeal obstruction (usual snoring).

Multi-system atrophy is a rare condition producing multiple neurological abnormalities. Patients sometimes present with Parkinsonian-like symptoms (the probable cause of the patient 'slowing up'), and an autonomic neuropathy (hence the postural hypotension, bladder problems unresponsive to prostatectomy, impotence and absent sweating). On formal testing, his systolic BP fell 35mmHg on standing, and his diastolic fell 25mmHg, with no perceptible rise in pulse rate.

The stridulous breathing at night, either continuous or frank obstructive sleep apnoea, is due to a specific atrophy and weakness of laryngeal abductors. Sometimes the stridor is evident during wakefulness, or can be provoked by a rapid inspiration or exercise. The brainstem nuclei supplying these muscles seem to degenerate early. With the general loss of muscle tone occurring at sleep onset, the larynx may critically narrow. Sudden nocturnal death is reported in this condition, and fatal closure of the larynx is postulated. Continuous positive airway pressure (CPAP) works in this condition and is able to splint open the cords. Thus CPAP should probably be offered, even if daytime sleepiness is not troublesome. Alternative surgical solutions, such as an arytenoidectomy or tracheostomy, are available.

In addition he had features to suggest REM sleep behaviour disorder (when dreams are physically acted out). REM behaviour disorder is also a feature of both Parkinson's and Shy–Drager syndrome, occurring when the area of the brainstem responsible for paralysing most muscles during REM sleep (Jouvet's centre) is damaged, thus allowing the motor activity associated with dreaming to be reflected in muscle activity. This varies from a general waving about of the arms and legs with shouting, through to highly aggressive and dangerous behaviour, often centred on fighting off attackers in the dream. REM behaviour disorder is also seen in some other brain degenerative disorders such as dementia with Lewy bodies.

During a sleep study, with video, it may be obvious that there are abnormal movements and shouting. If these are not overt during the sleep study, then a polysomnographic study may demonstrate an attenuation of the normal degree of dropout of submental EMG activity during REM sleep. REM behaviour disorder can occur many years before the features of Parkinson's or Shy–Drager syndrome declare themselves.

Progress

CPAP was initiated with full resolution of the stridulous breathing at night and partial improvement of the ESS (to 11/24). Clonazepam suppressed the REM behaviour disorder, but the other symptoms of multi-system atrophy have continued to progress.

Further reading

Chokroverty S (1996). Sleep and degenerative neurologic disorders. *Neurol Clin*; **14**: 807–826.

Case 15

A 51-year-old man was referred with bouts of coughing followed by syncope. He described one initial episode of syncope following a sudden bout of coughing 18 months previously, and had been free of symptoms until 3 months ago. He described a persistent cough most days, not worse at any particular time of day or night (not wakening him at night) and not associated with any other respiratory, nasal or reflux symptoms. He had two or three episodes each week, where he rapidly lost consciousness following a few short coughs; this included one episode when he was driving his Heavy Goods Vehicle (as a refuse collector for the local council). He had never smoked, and had been taking citalopram for mild depression, and lisinopril for hypertension for the last 3 years. Full cardiovascular, respiratory and neurological examinations were normal. CXR and spirometry were also normal.

Questions

15a) How would you further investigate and manage this patient?

15b) What is the pathophysiology of cough syncope?

15c) What advice would you give to this patient about driving?

Answers

15a) **How would you further investigate and manage this patient?**

The 2 key issues are managing the cough and the complicating factor, cough syncope.

The most important first step in managing this patient is the cessation of his ACE inhibitor. ACE inhibitors cause cough through excess bradykinin production, which sensitizes the cough reflex. Cough can develop even years after starting treatment. Following cessation of ACE inhibitors, median time to cough resolution is about 4 weeks but often takes longer (up to 10 months has been reported). Continued use of ACE inhibitors makes management of cough related to an additional pathology particularly difficult. The patient must be switched to an alternative antihypertensive. Angiotensin II receptor antagonists do not provoke cough.

If the cough persists after an acceptable time off an ACE inhibitor (e.g. 3 months) then a management strategy for chronic cough is required.

The three most common causes of chronic cough (defined as cough >8 weeks duration), in the absence of *any* specific clues from either history, examination or baseline investigations (as in this case), are:

- asthma syndromes (cough variant asthma, eosinophilic bronchitis)
- reflux disease (gastro-oesophageal reflux, laryngo-pharyngeal reflux, oesophageal dysmotility) and
- sinonasal disease, e.g. allergic or non-allergic rhinitis, sinusitis (often termed post-nasal drip, PND) or upper airway cough syndromes (UACS).

The best way of establishing a precise diagnosis is usually with sequential trials of treatment, in combination with selected diagnostic testing. Peak flow monitoring to look for diurnal variability is worthwhile, but is usually normal in 'cough-variant' asthma. Histamine or methacholine challenge testing has high sensitivity for asthma, so may be helpful as a 'rule-out' test, but lacks specificity and will not rule out eosinophilic bronchitis. Ambulatory pH monitoring will not identify 'non-acid' reflux, but is helpful in the small proportion of patients who may ultimately be considered for surgical management of reflux (e.g. Nissen's fundoplication) where some form of pre-operative objective diagnostic information is advisable.

In a unit receiving referrals primarily from general practice, asthma would be the most common diagnosis, followed by reflux, then PND/UACS.

It is always possible that patients may have more than one contributing factor to their cough. Each therapeutic trial should last at least 3 months; some centres would argue for 6 months for reflux, with additional use of pro-kinetic agents, e.g. metoclopramide (10mg three times a day). A suggested therapeutic strategy is given in Fig. 15.1. Experience from specialist clinics suggests this approach can achieve improved symptoms in over 80% of patients. At each point in the process it is important to emphasize the importance of compliance and the need for patience (on both physician and patients' part!). Particular care is needed in ensuring patients are instructed on how to use any inhaler device and appropriate administration of topical nasal medication.

If such an approach is not successful, further investigation (e.g. HRCT, bronchoscopy) is warranted to look for the more unusual causes of cough (such as bronchiectasis or tracheal amyloid). In specialist clinics,

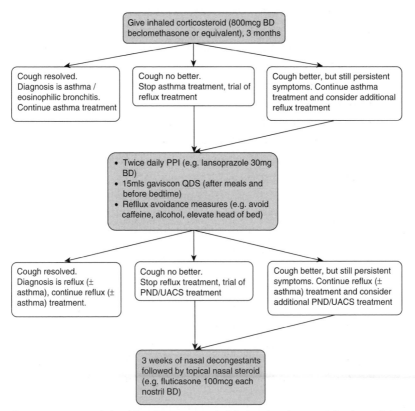

Fig. 15.1 Suggested algorithm for treatment trials for chronic unexplained cough in presence of normal CXR and spirometry.

up to 20% of patients may not have a cause for their cough identified (so called idiopathic chronic cough).

Treatment of cough syncope involves treatment of the underlying cause of the cough. There are no additional specific treatments for cough syncope, although atropine has been found to be effective in a single, blind, randomized controlled trial of patients with vasovagal syncope (Santini *et al.* 1999).

From the cough syncope point of view, investigations would include resting 12 lead ECG and referral for more prolonged ECG monitoring, given his occupation and Driver and Vehicle Licensing Authority (DVLA) regulations. A variety of cardiac electrophysiological abnormalities have been reported as causing cough syncope (sinus arrest, Mobitz II atrioventricular block, complete heart block) and permanent pacemaker insertion may be necessary if a significant bradyarrythmia is demonstrated.

15b) **What is the pathophysiology of cough syncope?**

The mechanism of cough syncope has been debated since its first description in 1876 by Charcot. There is no doubt that reduced intra-cerebral blood flow is the final common pathway for its occurrence, but how this results is not entirely clear, particularly if one is not able to demonstrate a bradyarythmia on continuous ECG monitoring that includes an event.

An early view proposed that, with prolonged coughing, the increased intrathoracic pressure reduced venous return to the heart and consequently a fall in the cardiac output, as occurs in a Valsalva manoeuvre. This was demonstrated in 27 patients with continuous coughing (Sharpey-Shafer 1953) but would not explain why syncope can occur after just a few coughs. A later view suggested that increased cerebral venous pressure, rather than reduced perfusion pressure, was to blame, whereby the increased intrathoracic pressure is transmitted to the cerebral circulation via the great veins with resultant decreased cerebral blood flow despite preserved arterial pressure (Mattle *et al.* 1995). This theory is contradicted by more recent work, which again comes down on the side of a neurally mediated reflex causing systemic hypotension, similar to an ordinary vaso-vagal event (Benditt *et al.* 2005). In this study, 9 patients with cough syncope were compared with two other groups: 13 syncope patients exhibiting a positive tilt test, and 18 patients with unexplained syncope. The cough syncope patients demonstrated a much greater fall in systolic blood pressure (median of 50mmHg) compared to the other two groups in response to two 'vigorous, volatile' coughs. This was accompanied by a blunted heart-rate response to the hypotension, and a slower recovery of blood pressure. It is not clear, however, how many of the patients, if any, actually had a syncopal attack during the study. If a neurally mediated reflex is to blame, there are a number of potentially responsible receptor sites (carotid, atrial or pulmonary baroreceptors).

15c) **What advice would you give to this patient about driving?**

Driving must stop immediately (both his heavy goods vehicle and his car). He must inform the DVLA of his diagnosis. If asystole is demonstrated on ECG monitoring, he may be considered fit to drive (HGV and car) once a pacemaker is inserted. If ECG shows no evidence of asystole, he must not drive until attack-free for 5 years. Cough syncope in HGV drivers has been reported as causing fatal accidents, with the drivers in each case avoiding prosecution (McCorry and Chadwick 2004). Interestingly this depended on a clear and consistent reporting of a characteristic history. The precise wording of DVLA advice for conditions relevant to respiratory and sleep medicine is shown in Table 15.1.

Table 15.1 DVLA advice for patients with respiratory conditions

Condition	Group 1 Entitlement (car, motorcycle)	Group 2 Entitlement (LGV/PCV)
Sleep disorders (including obstructive sleep apnoea syndrome, causing excessive daytime/awake, time sleepiness)	Driving must cease until satisfactory control of symptoms has been attained, confirmed by medical opinion	Driving must cease until satisfactory control of symptoms has been attained, with ongoing compliance with treatment, confirmed by consultant/specialist opinion. Regular, normally annual, licensing review required
Cough syncope	Driving must cease until liability to attacks has been successfully controlled, confirmed by medical opinion.	Driving must cease. If there is any chronic respiratory condition, including smoking, will need to be free of syncope/pre-syncope for 5 years. Individuals identified as having asystole in response to coughing can be considered once a pacemaker has been implanted and working

continued

Table 15.1 DVLA advice for patients with respiratory conditions *(continued)*

Condition	Group 1 Entitlement (car, motorcycle)	Group 2 Entitlement (LGV/PCV)
Carcinoma of lung	DVLA need not be notified unless cerebral secondaries are present.	Those drivers with non small cell lung cancer classified as T1N0M0 can be considered on an individual basis. In other cases, driving must cease until 2 years has elapsed from the time of definitive treatment. Driving may resume, providing treatment is satisfactory and no brain scan evidence of intracranial metastases
Narcolepsy/ cataplexy	Cease driving on diagnosis. Driving will be permitted when satisfactory control of symptoms achieved, then 1, 2 or 3-year licence with regular medical review	Generally considered unfit permanently, but if a long period of control has been established, licensing may be considered on an individual basis
Cerebral malignancy (including secondary deposits)	Normally, a period of 2 years off driving is required following treatment	Permanent refusal or revocation

Further reading

http://www.dft.gov.uk/dvla/medical/ataglance.aspx (accessed 1st September 2009)

Benditt DG, Samniah N, Pham S, Sakaguchi S, Lu F, Lurie KG *et al.* (2005). Effect of cough on heart rate and blood pressure in patients with 'cough syncope'. *Heart Rhythm*; **2**(8): 807–813.

Irwin RS, Curley FJ, French CL (1990). The spectrum and frequency of causes, key components of the diagnostic evaluation, and outcome of specific therapy. *Am Rev Respir Dis*; **141**: 640–647.

Mattle HP, Nirkko AC, Baumgartner RW, Sturzenegger M (1995). Transient cerebral circulatory arrest coincides with fainting in cough syncope. *Neurology*; **45**:498–501.

Morice AH, McGarvey L, Pavord I (2006). BTS guidelines: recommendations for the management of cough in adults. *Thorax*; **61** (Supp 1): 1–24.

McCorry DJP and Chadwick DW (2004) Cough syncope in Heavy Goods Vehicle Drivers. *Q J Med*; **97**: 631–632.

McGarvey LP, Heaney LG, Lawson JT *et al.* (1998). Evaluation and outcome of patients with chronic non-productive cough using a comprehensive diagnostic protocol. *Thorax*; **53**: 738–743.

Santini M, Ammirati F, Colivicchi F, Gentilucci G, Guido V (1999). The effect of atropine in vasovagal syncope induced by head-up tilt testing. *European Heart Journal*; **20**: 1745–1751.

Sharpey-Shafer EP (1953). The mechanism of syncope after coughing. *BMJ*; **2**: 860–863.

Case 16

A 37-year-old woman had several years' history of slowly progressive breathlessness, and a cough productive of small volumes of sputum. She had obstructive spirometry (FEV$_1$ 1.06L, 36% of predicted, and FEV$_1$/FVC ratio 38%) with no reversibility (FEV$_1$ improvement less than 15% after nebulized salbutamol). She had been on maximal therapy for asthma for several years. She was a smoker with an 18-pack year history, and worked as a shop assistant. Her father had died in his 50s from a respiratory condition.

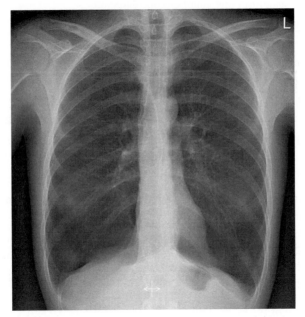

Fig. 16.1 CXR.

Questions

16a) What does her CXR show (Fig. 16.1)?

16b) Suggest the most likely cause for this lady's presentation, and some less likely alternatives that should be considered.

16c) Discuss the single investigation that could be carried out to diagnose the most likely condition.

Answers

16a) **What does her CXR show (Fig. 16.1)?**

Her CXR show hyperinflated lung fields with flattened diaphragms. There is increased basal lucency.

16b) **Suggest the most likely cause for this lady's presentation, and some less likely alternatives that should be considered.**

Causes of fixed airflow obstruction. This young lady is a smoker with fixed airflow obstruction, as illustrated by spirometry and CXR. With onset at this early age, a likely diagnosis is alpha-1 antitrypsin deficiency. Other diagnoses that could be considered are:

- Obliterative bronchiolitis (previous history of organising pneumonia or a connective tissue disorder?)
- Chronic asthma with chronic sub-optimal control (causing airways remodelling and loss of reversibility)
- COPD with increased risk-factor exposure (very early age of starting smoking? Occupational exposure? Concomitant cannabis smoking?)
- Upper airway obstruction due to a thyroid goitre or tumour, although the history of several years makes a tumour less likely (do airflow loops show predominant inspiratory airflow limitation?)

16c) **Discuss the single investigation that could be carried out to diagnose the most likely condition.**

A single investigation to diagnose alpha-1 antitrypsin deficiency is blood alpha-1 antitrypsin levels: normal range 20–52 mol/L (1.5–3.0g/L).

The patient in this case had serum alpha-1 antitrypsin levels of 2.4 mol/L (0.2g/L), well below both the normal range and the protective threshold of 35% of the normal mean value ($\leq$11 mol/L or $\leq$0.8g/L). Above this level, pulmonary symptoms tend not to occur. Her C-reactive protein (CRP), measured simultaneously, was not high. This is important as alpha-1 antitrypsin is an acute phase protein and can transiently increase, thus the test should be repeated if the CRP is high.

Questions

16d) What general pointers increase the likelihood of alpha-1 antitrypsin deficiency?

16e) Discuss the genetic basis of this condition.

16f) What is the mechanism of liver and lung disease in alpha-1 antitrypsin deficiency?

16g) What advice should this patient be given?

16h) What monitoring should she have?

Answers

16d) **What general pointers increase the likelihood of alpha-1 antitrypsin deficiency?**

Pointers suggesting the **possibility of alpha-1 antitrypsin deficiency:**

- Pulmonary emphysema in a young adult (<45y)
- Pulmonary emphysema with a modest smoking history or little exposure to dust or high concentrations of airborne particles
- Pulmonary emphysema, predominantly in the lower lobes
- Chronic hepatitis without another explanation
- Family members with pulmonary disease or ancestors with pulmonary emphysema in young adulthood, bronchiectasis or liver cirrhosis.

16e) **Discuss the genetic basis of this condition.**

Genetic basis of alpha-1 antitrypsin deficiency. The patient in this case was found to be homozygous for alpha-1 antitrypsin deficiency, ZZ.

- Inheritance: autosomal co-dominant
- Incidence: 1 in 2000–5000 (although significantly under-recognized)
- Gene: encoded by the SERPINA1 gene (formerly known as Pi), containing more than 100 allelic variants
- Classification: by the effects on serum levels of alpha-1 antitrypsin protein:
  - *M alleles* are normal variants, associated with normal alpha-1 antitrypsin levels; constitute 95% of those found in Caucasians
  - *S alleles* in homozygous form are associated with plasma alpha-1 antitrypsin levels of 60% normal, and are more frequent in the Mediterranean area
  - *Z alleles* in homozygous form are associated with plasma alpha-1 antitrypsin levels of 10–15% normal, and account for 95% of cases of severe deficiency
  - *The null allele* is associated with no detectable circulating alpha-1 antitrypsin, and is very rare
  - *Heterozygotes* with MS or MZ alleles have modestly reduced alpha-1 antitrypsin levels, but are not usually symptomatic.
- Gene frequency: alpha-1 antitrypsin deficiency is one of the most common genetic disorders to affect the white population, with 8% of Northern Europeans and 25% of the population of the Iberian Peninsula carrying an S- or Z- allele for alpha-1 antitrypsin. This has

led to speculation regarding a possible survival benefit. It has been postulated that, in the pre-antibiotic era, amplified inflammatory response might limit invasive respiratory and gastro-intestinal infection; since the availability of antibiotics, and widespread uptake of smoking, the pro-inflammatory properties of alpha-1 antitrypsin deficiency have on balance become detrimental.

16f) **What is the mechanism of liver and lung disease in alpha-1 antitrypsin deficiency?**

Alpha-1 antitrypsin is the antiprotease in the lung present in the highest concentration. It inactivates proteolytic enzymes in pulmonary tissue, most importantly neutrophil elastase in a ratio of 1:1, for which is has the highest affinity. Proteases are released into lung tissue during phagocytosis of airbourne pathogens. Without adequate clearance, such as occurs in alpha-1 antitrypsin deficiency, they remain active and slowly proceed to destroy the lung matrix components, alveolar structures and blood vessels. Within a few decades, the progressive destruction results in COPD. In addition to its antiprotease activity, alpha-1 antitrypsin may inhibit immune responses, stimulate tissue repair and matrix production, and have antibacterial activities.

Mechanism of disease in alpha-1 antitrypsin deficiency in the liver. In the liver in patients with the ZZ variant, further processing of alpha-1 antitrypsin protein synthesized in the rough endoplasmic reticulum of hepatocytes is delayed, so that approximately 85% of synthesized molecules polymerize into large conglomerates. These cannot be processed further and accumulate in the rough endoplasmic reticulum. Continued accumulation may result in cell injury and later in cell death. Patients have a highly increased risk of liver fibrosis and cirrhosis. Null variants synthesize no alpha-1 antitrypsin, and therefore have no liver disease.

16g) **What advice should this patient be given?**

In alpha-1 antitrypsin deficiency, the mean life-expectancy for smokers is 48–52 years, with disease progressing more quickly whilst smoking. For non-smokers, life-expectancy is nearly normal. She should, therefore, be advised to stop smoking, and blood relatives advised not to smoke (in particular of course any siblings who will have a 1 in 4 chance of alpha-1 antitrypsin deficiency for this autosomal recessive condition), with appropriate support offered to achieve this. Genetic counselling is not routinely offered at present, but may become indicated if specific therapy is developed in the future.

16h) **What monitoring should she have?**

Disease progression should be monitored with spirometry (or full pulmonary function tests), and liver function tests at intervals (annually is sufficient). Adults with alpha-1 antitrypsin deficiency develop liver disease less frequently than pulmonary manifestations. Hepatic symptoms manifest initially as hepatitis, followed later by fibrosis or cirrhosis. If abnormal liver function tests develop, the patient should be investigated further with a liver ultra-sound, screened for other causes of hepatitis or cirrhosis, and specialist hepatic referral may be appropriate. A small proportion of patients with homozygous deficiency genotypes develop neonatal hepatitis syndrome with cholestasis. This usually resolves after a few weeks, and is not associated with adult liver disease. Patients may be referred to a specialist centre; in the UK these are in Birmingham, Edinburgh and Cambridge.

Clinical progress

Following the diagnosis of alpha-1 antitrypsin deficiency with COPD, she discontinued smoking. Over the next 10 years her condition progressively worsened. She had recurrent infective exacerbations and a reduced exercise tolerance, with difficulty climbing hills, and was only able to climb half to one flight of stairs. Her FEV_1 was 1.1L (38% of predicted). She was on optimal therapy for COPD, including high-dose inhaled steroids, long- and short-acting beta agonists, and tiotropium. She had completed a pulmonary rehabilitation programme, and had pneumococcal and influenza vaccinations. A CT-chest of a patient with alpha-1 antitrypsin deficiency (not the patient in this case) is illustrated in Fig. 16.2.

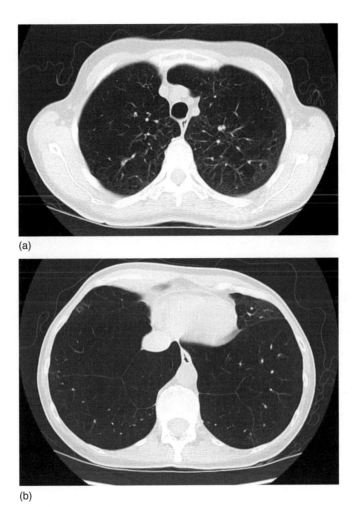

(a)

(b)

Fig. 16.2 CT chest.

Questions

16i) What features of alpha-1 antitrypsin deficiency does the CT-scan (Fig. 16.2) illustrate?

16j) What further treatent specific to alpha-1 antitrypsin deficiency may become available in the future?

Answers

16i) **What features of alpha-1 antitrypsin deficiency does the CT-scan (Fig. 16.2) illustrate?**

The CT scan shows predominant basal disease, with pan-acinar emphysema. Associated bronchiectasis is commonly seen, although not present in this case.

16j) **What further treatment specific to alpha-1 antitrypsin deficiency may become available in the future?**

No treatment specific to alpha-1 antitrypsin is currently recommended. At present treatment simply consists of optimization of usual COPD therapies, including smoking cessation, and in severe end-stage disease, consideration of lung transplantation in carefully selected patients.

'Augmentation therapy' with alpha-1 antitrypsin supplementation has been trialled, with a target serum alpha-1 antitrypsin level of 11μM or greater, since this level protects from development of emphysema. This level was achieved in one trial with weekly intravenous alpha-1 antitrypsin at a dose of 60mg/kg from pooled human plasma, without significant adverse events. Subsequent studies have trialled different doses and time intervals. Studies are inconclusive with some, but not all, showing a modest reduction in rate of decline of FEV_1, one showing a mortality benefit, and another a trend towards slower loss of lung tissue on CT. Benefits were seen in patients with moderate severity COPD only.

A recent 2½-year study (Dirksen *et al.* 2009) of weekly intra-venous alpha-1 antitrypsin in 77 patients has shown a significant reduction in exacerbation severity, but only a trend towards reduction in exacerbation frequency and reduced progression of disease on CT of the chest.

Augmentation therapy using inhaled alpha-1 antitrypsin has been considered, and demonstrated to increase concentrations in the epithelial lining fluid. Adequate delivery to the periphery of the lungs and to the interstitium remains a challenge, especially as many patients with deficiency already have abnormal lungs with heterogeneous ventilation.

Augmentation therapy confers no benefit to patients with liver disease, since pathogenesis relates to accumulation of unsecreted alpha-1 antitrypsin within hepatocytes.

Trials of other strategies may be undertaken in the future, e.g. use of inhaled recombinant secretory leuko-proteinase inhibitor, gene therapy to transfect airway cells with the alpha-1 antitrypsin gene or strategies to facilitate liver secretion of the Z variant of alpha-1 antitrypsin by preventing its polymerization or use of chaperone molecules.

Further reading

Abusriwil H, Stockley RA (2006). Alpha-1 antitrypsin replacement therapy: current status. *Curr Opin Pulm Med*; **12**: 125–131.

Dirksen A, Piitulainen E, Parr DG, Deng C, Wencker M, Shaker SB *et al.* (2009) Exploring the role of CT densitometry: a randomised study of augmentation therapy in alpha-1 antitrypsin deficiency. *Eur Respir J*; **33**:1345–53.

Heresi GA, Stoller JK (2008). Augmentation therapy in α-1 antitrypsin deficiency. *Expert Opin Biol Ther*; **8**: 515–526.

Kohnlein T, Welte T (2008). Alpha-1 antitrypsin deficiency: pathogenesis, clinical presentation, diagnosis, and treatment. *The Am J of Med*; **121**: 3–9.

Lomas DA (2006). The selective advantage of α-1 antitrypsin deficiency. *Am J Respir Crit Care Med*; **173**: 1072–1077.

Case 17

A 62-year-old man, with a history of pulmonary sarcoidosis, attended with progressive breathlessness over the preceding 6 months, such that current exercise tolerance was only 50 yards. In addition he had noticed increasing ankle swelling over the last 4 weeks. He denied any other respiratory or systemic symptoms and was a non-smoker.

His diagnosis of sarcoidosis was made 3 years previously following presentation (Table 17.1 PFT 1) with dyspnoea, and CT findings of diffuse ground glass with ill-defined centrilobar ground glass nodules. Because the appearances were atypical for sarcoidosis, a surgical lung biopsy was performed, which showed numerous discrete non-caseating granulomas in a perivascular and peribronchiolar distribution. There was patchy lymphocytic infiltrate, paucity of eosinophils and minimal fibrosis. Overall the appearances favoured sarcoidosis over alternative diagnoses. Following the lung biopsy, he was commenced on 40mg prednisolone, which improved his breathlessness (Table 17.1 PFT 2). Over the next 2 years his steroid dose was gradually tapered down to 5mg/day, but when seen at that point (Table 17.1 PFT 3), the dose was increased to 20mg as his dyspnoea had worsened. He had remained on this dose until he re-presented 9 months later (Table 17.1 PFT 4).

His past medical history included localized prostate carcinoma (treated with radiotherapy and hormonal treatment) and a monoclonal gammopathy of unknown significance (MGUS). On examination, resting SaO_2 on air was 88%, there was gross pitting oedema to the knees and the JVP was markedly elevated with prominent V waves. Cardiovascular examination revealed a marked right ventricular heave and a loud second heart sound. No murmurs were audible, and respiratory examination was otherwise unremarkable.

Investigations

- Hb 15.4g/dL, WCC 8.63 × 10^9/L (normal differential), platelets 158 × 10^9/L
- ESR 5mm/h, CRP 17mg/L
- U&E normal
- Bilirubin 27μmol/L, ALT 40IU/L, γGT 122IU/L, ALP 318IU/L
- Adjusted calcium 2.37mmol/L, ACE 35IU/L
- PSA <0.1ng/mL
- IgG paraprotein 9.3g/L (measured at 14g/L in 2005)
- IgM 0.13g/L (0.4–2.5), IgG 14.2g/L (6.0–13), IgA 1.7g/L (0.8–3)
- Urine electrophoresis normal, ANA, RF negative.

Table 17.1 Pulmonary function tests (serial values, with % predicted in parentheses)

Date	PFT 1	PFT 2	PFT 3	PFT 4
$FEV_1(L)$	3.2 (101)	3.5	3.0	2.5 (81)
FVC(L)	4.2 (103)	4.7	4.6	3.9 (99)
$FEV_1/FVC(\%)$	73	71	65	62
RV(L)	2.2 (90)	2.4	n/a	2.0 (83)
TLC(L)	6.2 (97)	6.1	n/a	5.9 (87)
VA(L)	5.4 (79)	5.8	6.1	5.5 (81)
TL_{CO}(mmol/min/kPa)	4.19 (45)	4.42	3.65	3.38 (37)
K_{CO}(mmol/min/kPa/L)	0.78 (57)	0.75	0.6	0.6 (47)

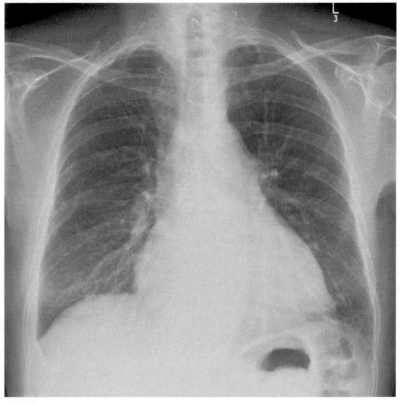

Fig. 17.1 CXR.

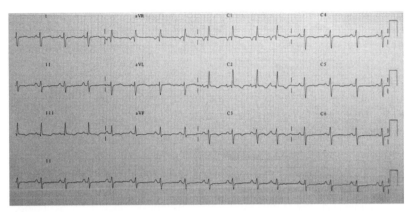

Fig. 17.2 ECG.

Questions

17a) What alternative diagnoses would have been considered at initial presentation in 2005 based on the radiological and pathological descriptions?

17b) Interpret the lung function tests, CXR (Fig. 17.1) and ECG (Fig. 17.2).

17c) What is the clinical diagnosis and what particular underlying causes should be considered?

17d) Give two key investigations that must now be performed.

Answers

17a) **What alternative diagnoses would have been considered at initial presentation in 2005 based on the radiological and pathological descriptions?**

Hypersensitivity pneumonitis, non-specific interstitial pneumonitis (NSIP) and respiratory bronchiolitis–interstitial lung disease (RBILD).

The radiological description of diffuse ground glass opacification with centrilobar ground glass nodules is, along with air trapping on expiratory CT slices (not seen in our patient), characteristic of hypersensitivity pneumonitis (HP; see case 8). HP is also a cause of non-caseating granulomata on lung biopsy, but the distribution described in the lung biopsy is more in keeping with sarcoidosis. On CT, sarcoid can cause diffuse ground glass but this is less common than the characteristic parenchymal finding of bronchovascular and fissural nodularity. NSIP can cause diffuse ground glass on CT but granulomas on biopsy are not a feature (see case 42). RBILD, which causes centrilobular nodules, ground glass opacification and also air trapping, could have been considered on radiological grounds but this is a disease of smokers.

17b) **Interpret the lung function tests, CXR (Fig. 17.1) and ECG (Fig. 17.2).**

The principle abnormality on lung function testing is a moderate reduction in gas transfer, which has significantly progressed (>10%) over time. There does appear to have been a reduction in FEV_1 over time, with the development of mild airflow obstruction (which might be a manifestation of peri-bronchiolar infiltration, although a reticular pattern on HRCT has been shown to correlate best with the degree of airflow obstruction). FVC and static lung volumes have not really changed over the course of the patient's attendance, which would have been expected if worsening fibrosis was the explanation. In sarcoidosis, parenchymal changes can progress initially without significant changes in FVC.

The CXR (Fig. 17.1) shows increased cardiothoracic ratio and a small right pleural effusion, but the lung fields and mediastinal contours are unremarkable. The ECG (Fig. 17.2) shows sinus rythm with right axis deviation and right ventricular hypertrophy (dominant R wave in V1, deep S waves V4–6)

17c) **What is the clinical diagnosis and what particular underlying causes should be considered?**

Pulmonary hypertension (PH). The main causes to consider in this patient are sarcoidosis as a direct cause, and thrombo-embolic disease.

17d) **Give two key investigations that must now be performed.**

 ◆ CTPA. The patient has underlying, albeit localized, prostatic malignancy, which would put him at risk for the development of pulmonary emboli and chronic thromboembolic pulmonary hypertension (CTEPH).

 ◆ Echocardiogram. To confirm the diagnosis and degree of PH, and to exclude left heart disease or intracardiac shunting as a contributory factor to the PH.

Further investigation

Echo confirmed PH with estimated pulmonary artery systolic pressure of >100mmHg. Right ventricular systolic function was severely impaired. There was right atrial enlargement, with tricuspid regurgitation. The left heart was normal in appearance with normal left ventricular systolic function and no evidence of any intracardiac shunts. A small pericardial effusion was seen.

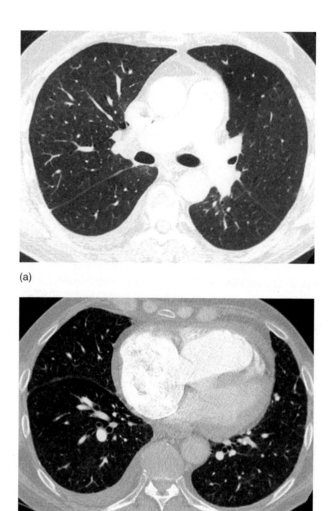

(a)

(b)

Fig. 17.3 CTPA.

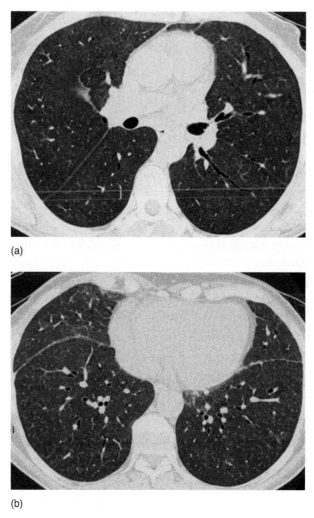

(a)

(b)

Fig. 17.4 Selected cuts from CT of 2005 for comparison.

Questions

17e) What are the key abnormalities on the CTPA and how does this examination differ from that of 2005?

17f) What action and further investigations are now required?

17g) Give five mechanisms by which sarcoidosis can cause PH.

Answers

17e) What are the key abnormalities on the CTPA and how does this examination differ from that of 2005?

The main findings on the CTPA are of pulmonary hypertension—the main pulmonary trunk is enlarged (Fig. 17.5), as are the left and right pulmonary artery. As a consequence of this, there is right ventricular and atrial enlargement. Not shown is tricuspid regurgitation with reflux of contrast into the inferior vena cava. There is also a small pericardial and a right pleural effusion. There is also a very subtle mosaic perfusion appearance to the lung fields (Fig. 17.5). No evidence of either acute or chronic thrombo-embolic disease was seen. Finally, no hilar or mediastinal lymphadenopathy was demonstrated. In comparison to the scan from 2005, the diffuse ground glass change has all resolved (there is much greater contrast between the major airways and parenchyma in the 2005 compared with current scan–the black bronchus sign). The diffuse centrilobar nodules have also resolved. The current CT, therefore, shows no evidence of active parenchymal sarcoidosis.

17f) What action and further investigations are now required?

Referral to a pulmonary hypertension centre is now needed for cardiac catheterization studies and consideration of specific therapy for PH. The precise cause of the patients PH is not clear at this point. Sarcoidosis remains a possibility but the patient now requires full investigation to exclude alternative causes of PH. Further investigations that could be organized pending review in a PH centre would be:

- V/Q scan. Although the CTPA shows no central or segmental emboli, in unexplained PH a Q scan is performed as a more sensitive measure of peripheral embolic disease.

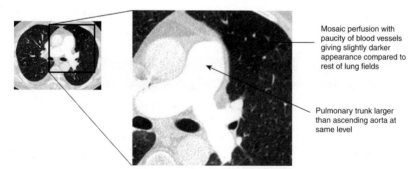

Mosaic perfusion with paucity of blood vessels giving slightly darker appearance compared to rest of lung fields

Pulmonary trunk larger than ascending aorta at same level

Fig. 17.5 Detail of CTPA image.

- Abdominal ultrasound. To exclude porto-pulmonary hypertension (development of pulmonary hypertension in association with portal hypertension from cirrhosis).
- HIV test. Pulmonary hypertension is a rare (1%) complication of HIV infection.

17g) **Give five mechanisms by which sarcoidosis can cause PH.**

Mechanisms by which sarcoidosis can cause pulmonary hypertension include:

- Progressive pulmonary fibrosis
- Secondary respiratory failure
- Compression of pulmonary arteries by lymphadenopathy
- Primary vasculopathy
- Pulmonary veno-occlusive disease.

The development of PH in sarcoidosis is usually attributed to fibrosis and destruction of pulmonary vessels in association with progressive parenchymal fibrosis (+/– contribution from chronic hypoxaemia). Development of pulmonary hypertension at the level of large pulmonary arteries can unusually occur with compression by lymphadenopathy. Diastolic dysfunction caused by myocardial sarcoidosis has also been reported as a cause of pulmonary venous hypertension.

In the absence of significant interstitial fibrosis, PH can arise from a primary vasculopathy where there is a granulomatous vasculitis involving veins and arteries to a varying extent. In one autopsy study of 40 patients (Takemura *et al.* 1992), the degree of granulomatous vascular involvement related to the degree of parenchymal granulomas, and venous involvement was more prominent than arterial involvement. Determining the mechanism of PH in patients without advanced fibrosis is often difficult without pathological examination of either large biopsies or autopsy specimens of explanted lungs. One series examined 22 patients with sarcoid and PH retrospectively (after exclusion of CTEPH). Fifteen had stage IV disease and seven had no fibrosis but did have more ground glass attenuation on CT than the fibrotic group. Five of the fifteen with severe fibrosis underwent lung transplantation. Four out of five had evidence of vascular granulomas (predominantly venous, and arterial granulomas seen only in two). In addition, an occlusive venopathy was seen in all five patients with intimal fibrosis, recanalization, chronic haemosiderosis and iron deposits on elastic laminae, in the absence of any other cause of pulmonary venous hypertension. The possibility of more than one causal mechanism inducing PH in the same patient, therefore, makes attributing degrees of causality difficult.

Progress

Unfortunately the patient collapsed and died at home before further investigations were performed. Post-mortem examination revealed massive pulmonary thrombo-embolism and evidence of extensive thrombus in the right iliofemoral vein. Unfortunately no lung tissue was retained for further histological assessment.

Further reading

Nunes H, Humbert M, Capron F, Brauner M, Sitbon O, Battesti JP (2006). Pulmonary hypertension associated with sarcoidosis: mechanisms, haemodynamics and prognosis. *Thorax*; **61**(1): 68–73.

Shigemitsu H, Nagai S, Sharma OP (2007). Pulmonary hypertension and granulomatous vasculitis in sarcoidosis. *Current Opinion in Pulmonary Medicine*; **13**: 434–438.

Takemura T, Matsui Y, Saiki S, Mikami R (1992). Pulmonary vascular involvement in sarcoidosis: a report of 40 autopsy cases. *Human pathology*; **23**(11): 1216–1223.

Case 18

A 48-year-old Caucasian woman presented to her general practitioner with dyspnoea on minimal exertion. She was wheezy on examination, peak flow was 210L/min (predicted = 470) and she was therefore diagnosed with asthma and started on inhaled β2 agonist and inhaled steroid. Despite this, she continued to deteriorate, but responded well to a short course of oral steroids. She was started on a combined high-dose steroid and long-acting β2 agonist inhaler, and provided with inhaler technique education. On review 1 month later, her peak flows had stabilized at around 370L/min and an asthma treatment plan was drawn up with the patient.

Four months later, she presented to the acute medical take with progressive deterioration over a 2-month period, requiring recurrent short courses of steroids from her GP. There was a 3-week history of productive cough, malaise and sweats. On examination, she was tachycardic, tachypnoeic and had widespread inspiratory crackles and cervical lymphadenopathy. SaO_2 on air was 90%.

Investigations

- Renal and liver function normal
- CRP >180mg/L
- Hb, 13.9g/dL, platelets, 672×10^9/L
- White cell count, 27.9×10^9/L (eosinophils 15.4×10^9/L)
- Urine dipstick negative for blood/protein
- CXR (Fig. 18.1), HRCT (Fig. 18.2).

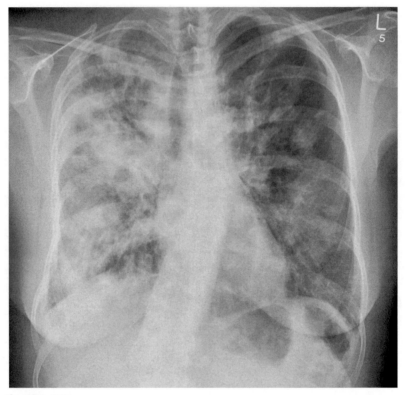

Fig. 18.1 CXR.

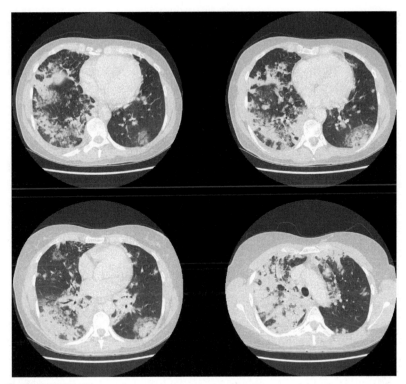

Fig. 18.2 HRCT chest.

Questions

18a) Describe the CXR.

18b) Provide a differential diagnosis for the CXR appearance.

18c) Provide a differential diagnosis for this case.

18d) Describe the HRCT images.

18e) What is the most likely diagnosis here and why?

18f) What investigations are indicated, and what is the management of this condition?

Answers

18a) **Describe the CXR.**

The CXR shows extensive patchy consolidation throughout the right lung field, small areas of consolidation with multiple nodules in the left-upper zone, and more extensive patchy consolidation in the left-lower zone. In addition there is a mild thoracic scoliosis.

18b) **Provide a differential diagnosis for the CXR appearance.**

The differential diagnosis of multifocal consolidation on the CXR includes the following:

Common causes

- ◆ Infection
  - Bacterial pneumonia
  - *Pnuemocystis jirovecii* pneumonia
  - TB (usually reactivation of latent disease)
  - Viral pneumonia (e.g. influenza)—more commonly diffuse or multifocal
- ◆ Neoplasm
  - Lymphoma (usually associated with hilar and mediastinal lymphadenopathy)
  - Broncho-alveolar cell carcinoma (rarely associated with hilar and mediastinal lymphadenopathy)
  - Multiple pulmonary metastases
- ◆ Inflammatory/other
  - Drug reactions (methotrexate, nitrofurantoin, amiodarone)
  - Parasitic disease (migration of *Ascaris* and *Strongyloides* nematodes through the pulmonary vascular bed)
  - Acute and chronic eosinophilic pneumonia
  - Cryptogenic organizing pneumonia (COP)

Uncommon causes

- ◆ Fungal pneumonias (blastomycosis, coccidioidomycosis)
- ◆ Melioidosis (consider in traveller to South East Asia)
- ◆ Septic pulmonary emboli (e.g. staphylococcal bacteraemia)
- ◆ Invasive aspergillosis (immunocompromised)

- ◆ Sarcoidosis
- ◆ Churg Strauss syndrome/Wegener's disease
- ◆ Collagen vascular disease (SLE pneumonitis, mixed connective tissue disease)
- ◆ Silicosis/pneumoconiosis (late stage).

18c) **Provide a differential diagnosis for this case.**

Eosinophilic lung disease may be associated with peripheral blood eosinophilia, or infiltration of the lung parenchyma with eosinophils with a normal peripheral count. Loeffler's syndrome (as in this case) is the association of lung infiltrates and a peripheral blood eosinophilia. The differential diagnosis for eosinophilic lung disease is as follows:

- ◆ Pulmonary eosinophilia
  - • Drug induced (e.g. nitrofurantoin, phenytoin)
  - • Acute eosinophilic pneumonia (AEP)
  - • Chronic eosinophilic pneumonia (CEP)
  - • Churg Strauss syndrome
  - • Allergic bronchopulmonary aspergillosis
  - • Asthma (usually mild eosinophilia)
  - • Parasitic infections: allergic reaction (*Ascaris*, hookworm, *Strongyloides*); parenchymal invasion (e.g. paragonomiasis); disseminated parasitic infection (e.g. schistosomiasis, *Strongyloides*); tropical pulmonary eosinophilia (*Wucheria bancrofti*, *Brugia malayi*)
  - • Other causes: idiopathic hypereosinophilic syndrome (HES); interstitial lung disease; neoplasia (including squamous cell lung carcinoma).

18d) **Describe the HRCT images.**

The HRCT shows multifocal bilateral consolidation (with air bronchograms) in the right-upper and lower lobes, and in the left-lower lobe. In addition, there is interlobar septal thickening in the right lung (Fig. 18.3).

18e) **What is the most likely diagnosis here and why?**

The most likely diagnosis is chronic eosinophilic pneumonia (CEP), which presents with cough, dyspnoea and systemic symptoms progressing over several months. Patients may experience chest pain, night sweats, myalgia and haemoptysis. A peripheral blood eosinophilia is seen in 70% of cases, and raised inflammatory markers and thrombocytosis are usual. The CXR reveals alveolar shadowing with the classical

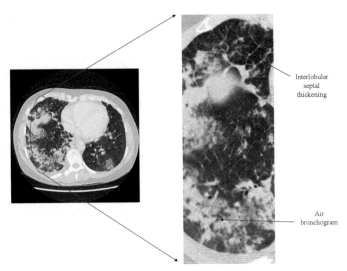

Interlobular
septal
thickening

Air
bronchogram

Fig. 18.3 Expanded HRCT chest.

description of 'photographic negative of pulmonary oedema' (extensive
bilateral peripherally based consolidation) seen in around 25% of cases.
Asthma is associated (either before or after the initial presentation) in
over 50%. Alternative possibilities include:

+ Acute eosinophilic pneumonia (AEP) is characterized by an acute
  illness (normally less than 7 days duration) associated with cough,
  dyspnoea, malaise, fevers and pleuritic chest pain. CXR reveals subtle
  interstitial infiltrates early in the disease, which may progress to florid
  consolidation that is not peripherally based. Small pleural effusions
  are common; peripheral blood eosinophilia is uncommon.

+ There is no travel history to suggest helminth disease

+ Although severe bilateral bacterial pneumonia or COP may produce
  this radiological pattern, a shorter history and more severe illness
  would be expected in bacterial pneumonia, and the typical 'migratory'
  pattern of COP is not demonstrated. In addition, such high peripheral
  eosinophil count is not expected in these conditions (and eosinopae-
  nia is expected during any systemic infection).

+ The absence of evidence of systemic vasculitis (upper respiratory tract,
  skin, peripheral nerves, heart, gut) makes Churg Strauss syndrome
  less likely.

+ Allergic bronchopulmonary aspergillosis is usually associated with
  central bronchiectasis and perihilar shadowing.

- In idiopathic hypereosinophilic syndrome (HES), a high peripheral blood eosinophilia (>1500/µl) for more than 6 months in the absence of identifiable cause is required for diagnosis, in association with organ involvement. Patients present with a chronic progressive systemic illness with weight loss, cachexia, pruritis and cough. Lung infiltrates are seen in up to one-third of cases, with the major morbidity and mortality associated with cardiac complications.

18f) **What investigations are indicated, and what is the management of this condition?**

Investigations:

- Authorities differ as to the level of investigation required to establish a diagnosis, with some suggesting lung biopsy as mandatory, while others suggest BAL is sufficient to exclude other diagnoses in association with a typical radiological pattern.
- BAL >40% eosinophils seen in CEP (>25% in AEP), excludes invasive helminth or fungal disease. In a case with convincing radiological and clinical features such as this, this may not be required.
- Lung biopsy may be undertaken where there is diagnostic doubt (characteristic histological features: interstitial and alveolar eosinophil infiltration, multinucleate giant cells, bronchiolitis obliterans with organizing pneumonia).
- Consider ANCA if Churg Strauss is a possibility, due to associated vasculitis (but p-ANCA positive in only 50% of Churg Strauss cases)
- IgE levels (>1000ng/mL), *Aspergillus* precipitins, aspergillus skin test if ABPA considered.

Management:

- Spontaneous recovery in CEP is rare (<10%), and continued illness may result in chronic respiratory impairment with irreversible fibrosis; therefore, prompt therapy is indicated once diagnosis is established.
- Oral steroid (prednisolone 40–60mg/day) titrated to eosinophil count (looking for total suppression)—CEP is highly sensitive to steroid treatment, and lack of response to steroid therapy should prompt reconsideration of the diagnosis.
- There are no randomized trials of therapy in CEP, but most authorities recommend continuation of high-dose therapy until, or for some weeks after, complete symptomatic and radiological resolution (4–6 weeks). Steroid dose should then be halved for 2 months.

- Total treatment course is recommended for between 3 and 9 months, as relapses are common. Dose should be tapered slowly, guided by clinical features, lung function and eosinophil count. Consideration should be given to bone protection therapy (calcium, vitamin D and a bisphosphonate) as long-term treatment is likely.
- In patients in whom decreasing steroid dose proves challenging, consideration should be given to alternate day regimens and steroid-sparing agents. There are case reports of success with high-dose, inhaled steroid, in addition to the lowest possible dose of oral prednisolone.
- In the case of disease relapse off therapy, steroid treatment should be re-initiated as above. The disease tends to respond well even after relapse. However, steroid therapy may be required for years, and some patients end up on permanent steroid therapy. The majority of patients (¾) require more than 19 months of therapy and some patients may require life-long therapy.
- In patients in whom deterioration occurs, evolution into Churg Strauss syndrome should be considered.

Progress

ANCA was negative. Bronchoalveolar lavage and transbronchial biopsies revealed evidence of eosinophilic pneumonia. The patient was commenced on prednisolone 30mg daily for 2 months, at which point slow tapering of the dose was attempted. Ten months later she was maintained on 10mg prednisolone per day with a normal eosinophil count, no symptoms and a normal chest radiograph. Rheumatological review suggested no evidence of vasculitis.

Further reading

Marchand E, Cordier JF (2006). Idiopathic chronic eosinophilic pneumonia. *Semin Respir Crit Care Med*; **27**(2): 134–141.

Case 19

Case A

A 48-year-old woman presented to the respiratory sleep clinic with a complaint of general non-specific tiredness, excessive sleepiness, and snoring. Her Epworth sleepiness score (ESS) was 17/24 (upper limit of normal = 9). A routine sleep history revealed no obvious cause for the sleepiness, although she was currently seeing a counsellor for depression. Sleep study was normal, apart from approximately 30 minutes of snoring. A diagnosis of depression-induced sleepiness and tiredness was made.

Two months later, she complained of altered vision in the temporal field of her right eye. An optician found an incomplete right superior temporal quadrantinopia.

An MRI was performed (Fig. 19.1).

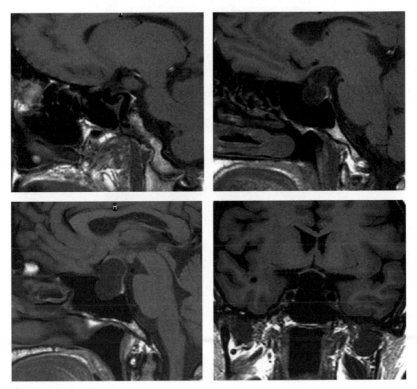

Fig. 19.1 Brain MRI.

Case B

A 40-year-old women was referred to the sleep clinic with an unusually rapid onset of sleepiness over 6 weeks. There were no features in the history, or on the sleep study, to suggest sleep apnoea, narcolepsy, periodic limb movements during sleep, poor sleep hygiene or depression. When alert, she was fully conscious and orientated.

A brain CT with contrast was performed (Fig. 19.2).

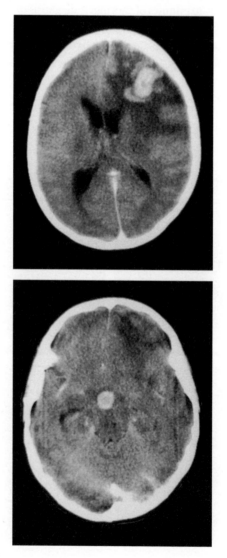

Fig. 19.2 Brain CT.

Questions

19a) What does the MRI on case A show?

19b) How could the lesion in the case A have been responsible for the earlier symptoms of tiredness and sleepiness?

19c) What does the CT show on case B?

19d) How could the lesions in case B have been responsible for the sleepiness?

Answers

19a) What does the MRI on case A show?

The MRI of case A shows a cystic lesion arising from, and expanding, the pituitary fossa with a significant suprasella extension. The chiasma and hypothalamus are significantly compressed. The appearances are of a Rathke's cleft (or pouch) cyst, a type of craniopharyngioma (Fig. 19.3).

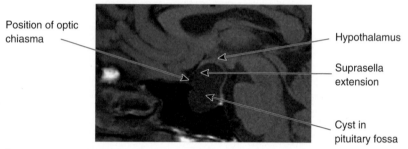

Position of optic chiasma

Hypothalamus

Suprasella extension

Cyst in pituitary fossa

Fig. 19.3 MRI, midline coronal section showing enlarged pituitary fossa.

19b) How could the lesion in the case A have been responsible for the earlier symptoms of tiredness and sleepiness?

This lesion might be causing the symptoms in two ways:

1. Pituitary function may be compromised with a consequent low cortisol. This patient had an entirely normal endocrine profile.

2. Compression of the hypothalamus and suprachiasmatic nucleus. The hypothalamus contains areas that control alertness/sleepiness and the supra chiasmatic nucleus is involved in controlling circadian rhythms.

Craniopharyngiomas are rare, usually suprasellar, and are either solid, cystic or mixed, benign tumours arising from remnants of Rathke's pouch along a line from the nasopharynx to the third ventricle. They are also known as Rathke's pouch tumours, hypophyseal duct tumors, or adamantinomas, depending on their histological type. They usually occur before age 20, or after age 40.

Sleepiness following surgical resection of, or radiotherapy to, craniopharyngiomas is also well-recognized, and is likely to be due to hypothalamic damage or altered levels of neurotransmitters (although secondary hormonal abnormalities do not seem to be the explanation).

19c) **What does the CT show on case B?**

The upper CT from case B (Fig. 19.2) shows a large enhancing, space-occupying lesion in the left-frontal lobe (with extensive surrounding oedema and midline shift). There is another enhancing lesion in the hypothalamus (centre of lower image, Fig. 19.2).

19d) **How could the lesions in case B have been responsible for the sleepiness?**

Again, involvement of the hypothalamus will also interfere with its function and potentially cause sleepiness.

Progress

In case A, surgical resection of the Rathke's cyst lead to resolution of the sleepiness, the Epworth sleepiness score falling to 9. In case B, left-frontal lobe biopsy revealed a B cell lymphoma; steroids, then radio-therapy, produced resolution of sleepiness and the patient is well 17 years later.

It is important in the sleep clinic to consider other diagnoses of excessive daytime sleepiness, apart from the common ones, such as sleep apnoea, poor sleep hygiene and depression. The following is a limited list of non-respiratory causes of sleepiness that may be encountered by those running a sleep clinic.

More common

- Depression, often missed
- Lifestyle issues/poor sleep hygiene—alcohol, late-night working, shift work, caffeine abuse, family circumstances, etc.
- Drugs—some of the anti-hypertensives (e.g. β blockers) and psychoactive drugs (e.g. anti-depressants and anxiolytics) can provoke sleepiness
- Narcolepsy—variable combination of cataplexy (sudden loss of muscle tone in response to excitement or anticipation), sleep paralysis (frightening paralysis on wakening for a few seconds or minutes) and prolific vivid dreaming, often at sleep onset
- Periodic limb movements during sleep (associated with restless legs during the day, especially in renal failure, and can be provoked by the SSRI anti-depressants)
- Simply being at the sleepier end of the normal spectrum.

Less common

- Hypothalamic damage (e.g. post-severe head injury, cranial irradiation or space-occupying lesion)

- Post-infectious (e.g. Epstein–Barr virus)
- Idiopathic hypersomnolence (sometimes hereditary)
- Certain neurological disorders, such as myotonic dystrophy, Parkinson's and previous stroke
- The symptom may really be tiredness, such as in 'ME' or insomnia, when the ESS is usually low, as this scale measures sleepiness rather than tiredness
- Insomnia/sleepiness in blind people with no retinal function—a circadian problem where the 24-h cycle is not linked with the real world through light and melatonin production.

Further reading

Chapman S, Robinson G, Stradling J, West S. (2009) Sleep and ventilation. *Oxford Handbook of Respiratory Medicine* (2nd edn), chapter 14, pp. 85–89.

Case 20

A 58-year-old man was referred with a fever up to 38°C associated with hepatitis, persisting despite several antibiotic courses. Investigations showed modestly elevated inflammatory markers (CRP, 75mg/L), a CXR showed pulmonary infiltrates, several sets of blood cultures, viral hepatitic screens and a myeloma screen were negative. Bronchoscopy was non-diagnostic. A liver biopsy showed caseating granulomas. His previous medical history included hypertension, prostatism and superficial transitional cell carcinoma of the bladder, treated with intravesical BCG (bacillus Calmette-Guérin) 8 months previously.

Question

20a) This patient's current presentation and urological history are related. Suggest an underlying diagnosis.

20b) How has the condition been acquired?

20c) What other clinical presentations are recognized?

Answers

20a) **This patient's current presentation and urological history are related. Suggest an underlying diagnosis.**

The underlying diagnosis is disseminated *Mycobacterium bovis*.

20b) **How has the condition been acquired?**

M. bovis has been acquired through intra-vesical BCG. BCG consists of live attenuated *M. bovis*. The mechanism of action of intra-vesical BCG is complex; it acts as a non-specific stimulant of the immune system by inducing granulomatous inflammation. Anti-tumour activity is concentrated at the site of BCG administration, hence topical application is used. Although virulence is markedly reduced, rarely it may cause infection or even dissemination after intra-vesical administration (1 of 200 in one case series) or BCG vaccination. Immunosupressed patients are much more susceptible to this. Intra-vesical BCG is widely used in the management of bladder cancer.

20c) **What other clinical presentations are recognized?**

Clinical presentation of *Mycobacterium bovis* infection. Symptoms can present within hours or up to years after intra-vesical BCG treatment. Clinical presentations include miliary pneumonitis, granulomatous hepatitis, soft tissue infections, bone marrow involvement and sepsis. Disseminated *Mycobacterium bovis* is a potentially life-threatening complication, and so clinicians must remain vigilant regarding its possibility even months or years after treatment.

Question

20d) Suggest other potential causes of fever post-intra-vesical BCG.

20e) What are the principles of treatment of *Mycobacterium bovis*?

20f) How are *Mycobacterium bovis* and *Mycobacterium tuberculosis* distinguished histologically and microbiologically?

Answers

20d) **Suggest other potential causes of fever post-intra-vesical BCG.**

The differential diagnosis of fever occurring post-intra-vesical BCG includes secondary Gram-negative sepsis and a hypersensitivity reaction. A much commoner side-effect of intra-vesical BCG is cystitis.

20e) **What are the principles of treatment of *Mycobacterium bovis*?**

If a patient is acutely unwell, and *Mycobacterium bovis* is suspected, as in this case, empirical therapy should be started before culture results are available. Choice of antibiotics for *Mycobacterium bovis* is similar to that for *Mycobacterium tuberculosis*; however, drug resistance is much commoner, in particular to pyrazinamide. In view of drug resistance, a longer duration of treatment of 9–12 months of all drugs, including at least rifampicin and isoniazid, is usually given. The patient had *Mycobacterium bovis* resistant to pyrazinamide and with intermediate resistance to isoniazid. He was treated with rifampicin, isoniazid, ethambutol and moxifloxacin for one year.

20f) **How are *Mycobacterium bovis* and *Mycobacterium tuberculosis* distinguished histologically and microbiologically?**

Mycobacterium bovis may cause caseating or non-caseating granulomas, whereas *Mycobacterium tuberculosis* usually causes caseating granulomas. Otherwise they are indistinguishable clinically or pathologically. Differentiation is only achieved following culture, and is suggested by the typical resistance pattern of *Mycobacterium bovis* to pyrazinamide.

Further case of *Mycobacterium bovis*

A retired agriculture lecturer had a lower respiratory tract infection that failed to respond to several courses of empirical antibiotics. His past medical history was of Crohn's disease, diagnosed 20 years previously. He had undergone a colectomy for refractory colonic and peri-anal disease. Colonic histology showed granulomas, initially thought to be non-caseating, supporting the diagnosis of Crohn's disease.

Given the failure of his lower respiratory tract infection to resolve, he underwent bronchoscopy, and was found to have *Mycobacterium bovis* infection. This led to re-examination of bowel histology from 20 years ago. In retrospect it was observed to show caseating granuloma, which would be consistent with a diagnosis of *Mycobacterium bovis* rather than Crohn's disease.

Question

20g) How might this man have acquired *Mycobacterium bovis*?

20h) What public health measures have led to reduced incidence of *Mycobacterium bovis* in the UK?

Answers

20g) **How might this man have acquired *Mycobacterium bovis*?**

The source of infection is not known for certain in this case; however, *Mycobacterium bovis* is a zoonosis that may infect humans, along with a broad range of domestic and wild mammals. Historically the commonest source has been from inhalation or ingestion of unpasteurized milk, which may have been the source in this case. Person-to-person transmission of *Mycobacterium bovis* is very rare.

20h) **What public health measures have led to reduced incidence of *Mycobacterium bovis* in the UK?**

Public health measures to reduce incidence of *Mycobacterium bovis* in the UK. Zoonotic TB was formerly an endemic disease in the UK due to consumption of raw cow's milk, with badgers helping to spread infection between herds of cattle. This has largely been eradicated by pasteurization of milk, and systematic culling of cattle reacting to compulsory tuberculin tests. Today most cases of zoonotic TB diagnosed in the UK are attributable to reactivation of long-standing latent infections acquired before widespread adoption of milk pasteurization, or *Mycobacterium bovis* infections contracted abroad.

Further reading

De la Rua-Domenech R (2006). Human *Mycobacterium bovis* infection in the United Kingdom: Incidence, risks, control measures and review of the zoonotic aspects of bovine tuberculosis. *Tuberculosis*; **86**: 77–109.

Paterson DL, Patel A (1998). Bacillus Calmette-Guerin (BCG) immunotherapy for bladder cancer: review of complications and their treatment. *Aust N Z J Surg*; **68** (5): 340–344.

Prescott S, Jackson AM, Hawkyard SJ, Alexandroff AB, James K (2000). Mechanisms of action of intra-vesical BCG. *Clin infection Dis*; **31 suppl 3**: S91–93.

Thoen C, LoBue P, de Kantor I (2006). The importance of *M bovis* as a zoonosis. *Vetinary Microbiology*; **112**: 339–345.

Case 21

A 52-year-old man with several years of snoring was referred for assessment of possible obstructive sleep apnoea. His wife described characteristic obstructive apnoeas during the night, increasingly frequent over the last year. The snoring had become so bothersome for the patient's wife that they often slept in separate rooms. The patient awoke feeling refreshed and did not complain of feeling sleepy during the day. He denied sleepiness on prolonged drives, was able to concentrate on reading a book and could watch TV for an hour or so in the evening without falling asleep. He had worked as a commercial airline pilot for the last 15 years and sleepiness had never interfered with his work. He had been successfully treated for essential hypertension for 12 years with bendrofluazide. On examination the patient had retrognathia, a collar size of 16 inches, BMI 25, normal nasal patency and no appreciable abnormality of the oropharynx. Completion of the Epworth sleepiness score (with wife present and agreeing with his account) gave a score of 3/24 (upper limit of normal, 9). A sleep study (Fig. 21.1) demonstrated severe obstructive sleep apnoea with an oxygen desaturation index (ODI >4% desaturations) of 58/h.

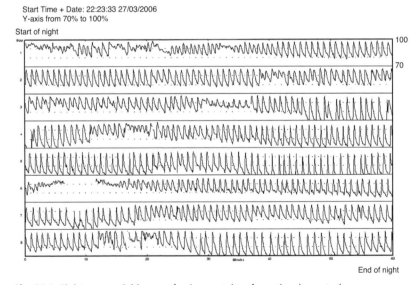

Start Time + Date: 22:23:33 27/03/2006
Y-axis from 70% to 100%

Start of night

End of night

Fig. 21.1 Eight sequential hours of oximetry taken from the sleep study.

Questions

21a) What treatment would you recommend for this patient?

21b) Would you undertake any further investigations?

21c) What advice would you give to this patient about driving?

21d) What impact will the diagnosis have on continuing employment as an airline pilot for this patient?

Answers

21a) **What treatment would you recommend for this patient?**

Although severe OSA was identified on sleep study, he does not complain of excessive daytime sleepiness and therefore does not have obstructive sleep apnoea <u>syndrome</u>. This distinction is important when deciding upon appropriate treatment, and when providing advice regarding driving (see answer 21c) and so on.

In the absence of excessive sleepiness, as long as there is no reason to think the patient is under-estimating this (corroborative history from partner is invaluable), there is little justification for recommending nasal CPAP. The principle reason for instituting CPAP in OSA is for the treatment of excessive daytime sleepiness. There is no convincing evidence that treatment with CPAP improves blood pressure control in non-sleepy patients with OSA, or indeed long-term morbidity or mortality. The patient (and his wife) are principally complaining of snoring and in the first instance careful enquiry as to potential aggravating factors (e.g. smoking, alcohol) should be undertaken. A jaw advancement device may be helpful in improving symptoms of snoring.

The patient must be counselled strongly that, if there is any concern about excessive daytime somnolence in the future, he must be re-assessed.

21b) **Would you undertake any further investigations?**

Further investigation in these circumstances would really depend on your belief as to the patient's true level of sleepiness, and whether you would wish to confirm this. There is not a good correlation between severity of OSA and level of sleepiness, but his OSA is severe and the Epworth sleepiness score may be purposely under-estimated if the patient (and their partner) fears he will lose his livelihood. In cases where either you do not believe the reported level of sleepiness, or you feel the patient needs convincing of their true level of sleepiness, a wakefulness test can help. These tests do not correlate with objective measures of severity of OSA (e.g. Apnoea-hypopnoea Index or ODI), or with future likelihood of a driving accident. In this case, however, because of his job as a pilot, objective clarification of his reported lack of sleepiness is recommended (see answer 21d).

Level of sleepiness can be more objectively defined by:

- Maintenance of wakefulness test (MWT). The patient is asked to stay awake lying semi-recumbent for 40 minutes in a quiet and darkened room on four occasions throughout the same day at 2-hourly intervals (again with continuous EEG monitoring) and length of time taken to fall asleep is recorded.

- Oxford sleep resistance test (OSLER). A variant of the MWT, except sleep latency is assessed behaviourally without EEG monitoring (and without a technician engaged in continuous monitoring of the EEG) and is, therefore, easier to administer. The patient is left semi-recumbent in a quiet and darkened room for 40 minutes, and is asked to stay awake and press a fingerpad in response to a dim light, lit regularly for 1 second in every 3. The number of missed responses is recorded, and persistent lack of response (failure to respond for 21 seconds, or 7 illuminations) defines sleep onset, recorded by computer.
- Multiple sleep latency test (MSLT). Conversely to the MWT, patients lie in a quiet, dim room and are asked to fall asleep (defined by EEG monitoring) on four or five occasions at 2-hourly intervals throughout the day and the time taken to do so is measured.

21c) **What advice would you give to this patient about driving?**

When considering driving, the over-riding principle, from a legal point of view, is that any patient who drives must take responsibility for being safe to drive. Any driver who falls asleep while driving and causes an accident involving themselves or others is personally liable and, in the case of fatal incidents, may be charged with causing death by dangerous driving, potentially receiving a gaol sentence. Patients with obstructive sleep apnoea syndrome must inform the DVLA of their diagnosis and not drive until established on treatment that has improved their excessive daytime sleepiness (see case 15). This patient, however, is adamant he is not sleepy and, therefore, does not need to inform the DVLA of his OSA diagnosis, as he does not have the syndrome. As long as he remains free of sleepiness, he can drive, but must be counselled strongly that, if the situation changes, he must not drive and be referred for re-assessment. All such patients should be advised not to drive if at all sleepy.

21d) **What impact will the diagnosis have on continuing employment as an airline pilot for this patient?**

He must inform his airline and the Civil Aviation Authority (CAA) of the diagnosis of OSA, but emphasize he does not have OSA syndrome. As with the driving rules, there should be no impact on his continuing to fly, but the CAA will require confirmation of lack of sleepiness by an objective measure. The same advice applies about needing re-assessment if sleepiness becomes a problem.

Were the situation different and sleepiness was a problem, a minimum of 6 weeks CPAP treatment, accompanied by improved sleepiness (ESS ≤9), is required before the CAA would allow such a pilot to fly. If there is any doubt then as to the genuine level of sleepiness, a MSLT is advised in current CAA guidelines, despite its poor ability to predict real life sleepiness and lapses in performance.

Further reading

http://www.caa.co.uk/docs/49/SRG_MedSleepApnoea.pdf (accessed 1st September 2009)

Bennett LS, Stradling JR, Davies RJO (1997). A behavioural test to assess daytime sleepiness in obstructive sleep apnoea. *J Sleep Res*; **6**: 142–145.

Stradling JR (2008). Driving and obstructive sleep apnoea. *Thorax*; **63**: 481–483.

Case 22

A 68-year-old man presented with 2 months of progressive breathlessness on exertion and weight loss of 7kg. He had a past medical history of an anterior myocardial infarction 3 months previously, and hypertension. He was a retired plumber and had had definite asbestos exposure in the past. He had never smoked.

On examination he had an oxygen saturation of 95% on air. There was dullness to percussion with reduced breath sounds audible over the left hemithorax.

Investigations

- Hb 14.3g/dL, WCC 10.7 × 10⁹/L, platelets 350 × 10⁹/L
- CRP 55mg/L
- U&E, LFT normal
- Pleural aspiration:
  - Serosanguineous fluid
  - Protein 51g/L, lactate dehydrogenase 869IU/L, glucose 3.5mmol/L, pH 7.27
  - Cytology negative
  - No growth on culture
  - CXR shown in Fig. 22.1.

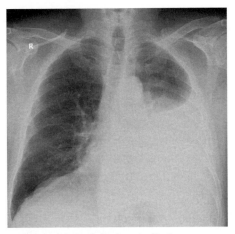

Fig. 22.1 CXR on presentation: large left pleural effusion.

Questions

22a) What are the differential diagnoses?

23b) What investigations would you perform next?

Answers

22a) **What are the differential diagnoses?**

Progressive breathlessness with a large pleural effusion is associated with many respiratory, and systemic, conditions. Measurement of protein and lactate dehydrogenase (LDH) should be requested on all initial pleural fluid aspirates, as determining whether the fluid is an exudate or a transudate usually further aids diagnosis (see Table 22.1).

Table 22.1 Causes of pleural effusion

Transudates	Exudates
Common	**Common**
Left ventricular failure	Parapneumonic effusion and empyema
Liver cirrhosis 'hepatic hydrothorax'	Malignancy
Hypoalbuminaemia	Tuberculosis
Peritoneal dialysis	Rheumatoid arthritis
Nephrotic syndrome	
	Less common
Less common	Pulmonary infarction
Hypothyroidism	SLE
Mitral stenosis	Other autoimmune diseases
Pulmonary embolism (10–20% transudates)	Benign asbestos-related pleural effusion (BAPE)
Constrictive pericarditis	Pancreatitis
Urinothorax	Post-cardiac injury syndrome (Dressler's)
Meigs' syndrome	Post-coronary artery bypass grafting
Superior vena cava obstruction	Hepatic/splenic/subphrenic abscess
Malignancy (up to 5% are transudates)	Oesophageal rupture
	Rare
	Ovarian hyperstimulation syndrome (may also be transudative)
	Yellow nail syndrome
	Chylothorax
	Drugs
	Sarcoidosis
	Fungal infections

In clinical practice, pleural fluid protein levels >35g/L represent an exudate, and <25g/L a transudate (if the patient has a normal serum protein concentration). However, Light's criteria can be applied in patients with intermediate protein values (i.e. 25–35g/L or abnormal serum protein); if any of the following criteria are met the fluid is an exudate:

+ Pleural fluid to serum protein ratio >0.5
+ Pleural fluid to serum LDH ratio >0.6
+ Pleural fluid LDH >2/3 the upper limit of normal serum LDH.

Caution should be taken, particularly with effusions in patients on diuretic therapy for heart failure, as although the underlying fluid is formed as a transudate, diuretics may result in an exudate on biochemical analysis through water removal (i.e. false-positives).

In this case, the pleural effusion was an exudate and the management strategy should focus on determining a cause from the list in Table 22.1.

Pleural effusions occur in up to 60% of patients with pneumonia. Clinically they represent a spectrum from (1) 'simple' parapneumonic effusion (reactive, sterile pleural fluid) to (2) 'complicated' parapneumonic effusion, with infected pleural fluid resulting in pleural fluid pH <7.2 and fibrinous septations, to (3) empyema—frank pus in the pleural space (or culture positive). In this case there were no clinical symptoms to suggest pleural infection, although these may not always be present, and an infective aetiology for his effusion is unlikely.

Malignant pleural effusions are responsible for approximately 22% of all pleural effusions. The progressive symptoms and weight loss raise concern of underlying malignancy including mesothelioma given his documented asbestos exposure.

Pleural effusions resulting from pulmonary emboli are typically small. In this case, the pre-test probability was low and few other clinical features (pleuritic chest pain or hypoxia) suggest this as a cause.

Dressler's syndrome (post-cardiac injury syndrome) is uncommon but should be considered. It usually arises 3–10 weeks after an acute myocardial infarction and presents with fever and pleuritic chest pain. Pleural effusions are commonly unilateral but may appear bilaterally. They result from an immunologically mediated reaction and a prompt response is seen with non-steroidal anti-inflammatory agents (NSAIDs) or corticosteroid treatment.

Drug-induced effusions should be considered and suspected culprits can be checked at: www.pneumotox.com (accessed 1st September 2009).

22b) **What investigations would you perform next?**

Next investigations:

(i) Thoracic CT with pleural phase enhancement would be an appropriate next investigation. In this case the CT appearances (Fig. 22.2) demonstrate a large pleural effusion with a rim of pleural thickening (arrows). These features suggest underlying malignant disease. CT can reliably differentiate benign from malignant pleural disease. Nodular (specificity 94%), circumferential (specificity 100%) pleural thickening with mediastinal extension (specificity 88%) and thickness >1cm (specificity 94%) are all characteristics of pleural malignancy, but not of the particular tumour type.

(ii) Cytological analysis of pleural fluid confirms the diagnosis of malignancy in 60% of cases. Analysis of a second sample may improve this rate by 27%, but further thoracenteses are not recommended. In this case, cytological diagnosis was not achieved. Pleural tissue for histological analysis should be obtained. Options include (1) imaging-guided pleural biopsy or (2) thoracoscopic biopsy, diagnostic sensitivity of malignancy is similar with both techniques. Blind pleural biopsy (i.e. Abram's) is not recommended for suspected malignant pleural disease (sensitivity 47% vs 87% with CT-guided biopsy technique in patients with definite pleural thickening).

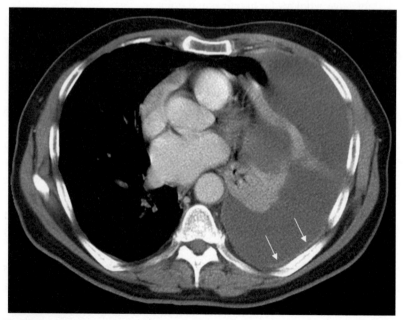

Fig. 22.2 CT chest.

Progress

Pleural biopsies performed under local anaesthetic thoracoscopy confirmed epithelioid malignant mesothelioma.

Questions

22c) What treatment options would you consider at this stage?

22d) What advice would you give the patient and his family regarding compensation and benefit claims?

22e) What is the prognosis?

Answers

22c) **What treatment options would you consider at this stage?**

Management of the patient with mesothelioma requires a multi-disciplinary approach and consideration of the following:

- ◆ Control of pleural effusion.

  Drainage of pleural fluid provides effective short-term symptomatic relief for most patients, but no data exist to predict which, or how quickly, effusions will recur (some reports, for all causes of malignant effusions, suggest up to 100% at 1 month, others a lower rate). Early definitive pleural intervention is, therefore, appropriate to reduce fluid re-accumulation, with fluid drainage and talc pleurodesis, either thoracoscopically or via a chest tube (success rate 60–90%). In some patients the lung fails to re-expand as a result of visceral tumour encasement ('trapped lung') and, as pleural symphysis is not possible in this group, attempts at pleurodesis is not recommended. Repeated pleural aspiration can be performed if symptoms persist and are relieved by fluid evacuation (this is also appropriate for patients in whom pleurodesis is unsuccessful).

  Insertion of an indwelling pleural catheter should be considered, if symptomatic pleural fluid re-accumulation necessitates continued repeat aspirations or hospital admissions, in patients with a reasonable performance status.

- ◆ Radiotherapy.

  Mesothelioma has a tendency to metastasize along tracts of previous pleural puncture sites. Prophylactic drain site radiotherapy has previously been shown to reduce tract spread but this finding was not confirmed in two recent randomized controlled trials. Its benefit remains a topic of debate. Radiotherapy is effective in treating tract metastases if they develop.

- ◆ Chemotherapy.

  The anti-folate drugs, pemetrexed (Alimta) and raltitrexed, in combination with cisplatin have been shown to improve life-expectancy (in the EMPHACIS trial, $n = 448$, median survival increased from 9.3 to 12.1 months with combination treatment compared to cisplatin alone ($P = 0.02$)). Although data are limited, single-agent pemetrexed has demonstrated promising activity in both chemo-naïve mesothelioma patients, and as a second line agent.

- ◆ Surgery.

  No quality evidence supports the use of radical surgery (extrapleural pneumonectomy, EPP) and this does not improve survival. It carries a high mortality (5–10%) and morbidity (25% life-threatening post-operative complications), and has recently been shown to significantly impair quality of life for at least 6 months post-operatively. The role of tri-modality treatment with EPP, adjuvant radiotherapy and chemo-therapy is under investigation. Large retrospective series have shown a worse prognosis for patients who underwent EPP, than for those who had pleurectomy/decortication (PD). A randomized trial on PD vs talc pleurodesis alone is underway.

- ◆ Psychological support.

  Involvement of the multi-disciplinary team is paramount to support patients and their carers. Patients with mesothelioma have unique psycho-social issues, such as the possible future need for a coroner's post-mortem, medico-legal aspects regarding compensation, specific fears of a 'horrible death' and resentment towards previous employers for lack of occupational protection.

- ◆ Pain control (see question 22f).

  Pain is a common symptom and regular analgesia is often required. Targeted radiotherapy can ease pain, e.g. from bone erosion or tract metastases. Percutaneous cervical cordotomy (interrupting the spi-nothalamic tract at C1-C2), application of intrathecal analgesia, or regional nerve blocks may be considered.

- ◆ Other.

  Anorexia and weight loss may be significant, and maintenance of a high-calorie diet should be advised. Oral corticosteroids may improve patients' appetite and sense of well-being. Complementary therapies, counselling and psychology input may help reduce feelings of anxiety and shock. Troublesome cough may ease with pleural effusion drain-age (see above), and use of a codeine, or simple linctus or oral opiate treatments, can be tried. Excessive sweating may be relieved using anti-pyretics, steroid therapy and anticholinergic agents. There is some evidence supporting thalidomide (by reducing cytokine pro-duction) but this should currently be for specialist use only.

22d) **What advice would you give the patient and his family regarding com-pensation and benefit claims?**

Application for compensation claims and benefit entitlements for asbestos-related disease can result in additional anxieties. Claims can be made for mesothelioma, asbestosis and diffuse pleural thickening; however, a recent ruling by the Court of Appeal (October 2007) has vetoed the rights of patients with pleural plaques to claim compensation.

It is worth involving a specialist solicitor early on, as direct evidence from the sufferer is valuable and more reliable than indirect recollections from the patient's next of kin.

For patients with mesothelioma, eligibility for compensation depends on demonstrating a clear history of occupational asbestos exposure. Patients should be given time to construct a detailed employment history, including companies worked for, duration and method of exposure, and any documentation (e.g. P60s, payslips) from the period of employment. The contact details of old colleagues who have also developed asbestos-related disease may be useful during the compensation process and allow corroboration of the exposure history.

Compensation claims may be sought from two main sources:

1. From the Government (Department of Work and Pensions (DWP), previously the DSS, 0800 882200).

    (a) Patients can apply for industrial injuries disablement benefit (IIDB) and are eligible for lump-sum payment (state compensation) under the Pneumoconiosis, etc. (workers' compensation) Act, but only if the IIDB claim is successful and they have not received payment via a common law action (see below).

If the patient is ineligible for Pneumoconiosis, etc. Act (workers') compensation they may be able to claim a one-off lump sum payment under the 2008 Diffuse Mesothelioma Scheme. This scheme covers people whose exposure to asbestos occurred in the United Kingdom and was not as a result of their work as an employee (e.g. those who were self-employed or had indirect exposure (i.e. via a relative or environmentally), or those who cannot trace their exposure).

    (b) If contact with asbestos was made when in the armed forces, a claim may be made via the war pension scheme. This is instead of industrial injuries disablement benefit (Veterans' Agency Helpline 08001692277)

2. Through the courts via common law (civil) proceedings against a previous employer. If the employer is still trading and/or the insurers are solvent, an experienced solicitor should be contacted. The Law Society (0870 6066575) or asbestos support groups (available via www.mesothelioma.uk.com, accessed 1st September 2009) have lists of specialist solicitors. If the former employers no longer exist, action may be taken provided the insurance company can be traced.

If the solicitor cannot find the employers or their insurers, patients may still be entitled to a lump sum payment under the Pneumoconiosis etc. Act (as above).

If patients have been solely self-employed, they are ineligible for benefit. This is uncommon and often a civil claim may be made through those with whom they were sub-contracted or did an apprenticeship with (although this would not assist entitlement to IIDB).

A 3-year 'statutory period from awareness of any asbestos-related disease' (including pleural plaques) exists for making a claim, although this 'limitation period' is not always strictly enforced.

Dependants of the patient may also take legal action to claim compensation. This can be initiated after the sufferer's death but must be done within 3 years. Accurate details of employment exposures can be difficult to obtain posthumously.

22e) **What is the prognosis?**

The prognosis of mesothelioma is poor with a median survival of approximately 9 months (although there are a small number of long term survivors >5 years).

Adverse prognostic factors include:

- Non-epithelioid (i.e. sarcomatoid or biphasic) histological subtype
- Poor performance status.

Weaker predictive factors of a poor outcome include:

- Presence of chest pain
- Age >75 years
- Male sex
- Elevated LDH, white cell and platelet counts
- Anaemia
- Weight loss.

Progress

Five months later the patient was seen in clinic and reported increasingly severe diffuse 'gnawing' left-sided chest pain, particularly at night. He was taking regular paracetamol and codeine with little relief.

Question

22f) How would you address this patient's pain?

Answer

22f) **How would you address this patient's pain?**

Pain may be secondary to diffuse pleural involvement, somatic pain (e.g. chest wall invasion) or neuropathic pain (e.g. intercostal nerve involvement). In this case, a repeat CT would assess disease progression. Options for pain relief include:

* Early use of opiate analgesia—rapid-dose escalation may be required
* Addition of NSAIDs
* Anticonvulsants (e.g. gabapentin, carbamazepine, sodium valproate) for neuropathic pain
* Radiotherapy for localized chest-wall pain (e.g. bony erosion, tract metastases)
* Percutaneous cervical cordotomy (interrupting the spinothalamic tract at C1/2 induces contralateral loss of pain sensation) performed in a specialist centre, has a low complication rate but patients should be warned about the risks of thermoanaesthesia, post-cordotomy dysaesthesia and unilateral motor weakness
* Use of cingulotomy for relief of refractory pain may be considered in selected patients, but is not easily available.

Further reading

Boutin C, Rey F, Viallat JR (1995). Prevention of malignant seeding after invasive diagnostic procedures in patients with pleural mesothelioma. A randomized trial of local radiotherapy. *Chest*; **108**: 754–758.

Garcia LW, Ducatman BS, Wang HH (1994). The value of multiple fluid specimens in the cytological diagnosis of malignancy. *Mod Pathol*; **7**: 665–668.

O'Rourke N, Garcia JC, Paul J, Lawless C, McMenemin R, Hill J (2007). A randomised controlled trial of intervention site radiotherapy in malignant pleural mesothelioma. *Radiother Oncol*; **84**: 18–22.

Robinson BWS, Lake RA (2005). Advances in malignant mesothelioma. *Lancet*; **353**: 1591–1603.

Vogelzang NJ, Rusthoven JJ, Symanowski J, Denham C, Kaukel E, Ruffie P *et al.* (2003). Phase III study of pemetrexed in combination with cisplatin versus cisplatin alone in patients with malignant pleural mesothelioma. *J Clin Oncol*; **21**: 2636–2644.

Case 23

An 88-year-old woman was admitted with a 6-month history of progressive shortness of breath, a cough productive of small volumes of clear sputum and lethargy. In the preceding 3 weeks her symptoms had worsened, also with episodes of feeling hot and shivery. Three courses of antibiotics from her GP had not improved symptoms. She had previously been given a diagnosis of late onset asthma, on the basis of several year's history of shortness of breath and wheezing at night, worse in the springtime and with exposure to oil seed rape. She had no other atopic history. Symptoms had improved a little with inhaled beclomethasone 200µg, two puffs twice daily and salbutamol, as required. She was an ex-smoker with a 10-pack year history.

She had a past medical history of hypertension, palpitations, congenital double uterus and absence of right kidney, recurrent cystitis, previous cholecystectomy, *Herpes zoster* infection and irritable bowel syndrome. Her long-term medications included diltiazem, furosemide, nitrofurantoin, omeprazole and mebeverin.

On examination she was dyspnoeic at rest, with a heart rate of 110 and respiratory rate of 32. She had bilateral inspiratory crackles, but no wheeze and no signs of fluid overload. Oxygen saturations were 89% on air.

Investigations

- Haemoglobin, 12.3g/dL
- White cell count, 14.1×10^9/L
- Neutrophils, 9.6×10^9/L
- Eosinophils, 1.1×10^9/L
- Platelets, 560×10^9/L
- U&E normal
- CRP, 58mg/L
- D-dimer, 1532µg/L (normal range <500)
- Troponin <0.02 (negative)
- Aspergillus (IgG), 1 precipitin line
- Aspergillus (IgE), <0.35kU/L (negative)
- Total IgE, 120kU/L (5–120)
- Anti-nuclear antibodies, 160 titre (0–80)
- ANCA negative
- Rheumatoid factor <9.5IU/ml (negative)

- ◆ ECG: sinus tachycardia, with normal axis, no ischaemic changes and first-degree heart block.
- ◆ Arterial blood gas on 28% FiO_2

pH	7.47
$PaCO_2$	4.5 kPa
PaO_2	11.2 kPa
SaO_2	97%
Base excess	1.0 mmol/L
Bicarbonate	26 mmol/L

- ◆ FEV_1/FVC ratio 83%.

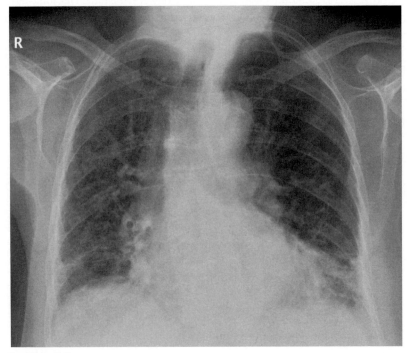

Fig. 23.1 CXR.

Questions

23a) Discuss potential causes of this lady's shortness of breath, with evidence for and against each.

23b) What step is important to try and halt the progression of her underlying condition?

Answers

23a) **Discuss potential causes of this lady's shortness of breath, with evidence for and against each.**

Possible contributors to her shortness of breath:

- Usual interstitial pneumonitis (UIP). This lady's history of shortness of breath, inspiratory crackles, restrictive spirometry, raised CRP and antinuclear antibodies, and infiltrates on CXR are in keeping with UIP. The deterioration over the preceding 3 weeks could have been caused by an accelerated phase of UIP, or by a co-existent condition, such as one of those listed below.

- Lower respiratory tract infection. An acute deterioration over 3 weeks may represent an infective cause. In support of this she had felt feverish, with raise acute inflammatory markers. The CXR is markedly abnormal, with reticular infiltrates and left basal opacification.

- Left ventricular failure. In support of this diagnosis she has cardiac risk factors (hypertension and a possible dysrhythmia); however, her ECG does not show acute ischaemic changes, and although the CXR shows an increased cardio-thoracic ratio, there are no Kerley-B lines or fluid in the lateral fissure to suggest heart failure.

- Pulmonary embolus. Several tests would support a diagnosis of pulmonary embolus, however, there are more likely causes for each of them. D-dimer is an acute-phase reactant, and so an elevated level is not necessarily indicative of thrombo-embolic disease in the presence of infection or an inflammatory disorder. She has a widened alveolar—arterial PO_2 gradient (PO_2 only 11.2kPa despite 28% inspired oxygen fraction); however, the presence of inspiratory crackles and CXR changes means there are other potential causes for this. The risk of pulmonary embolism is increased in congestive cardiac failure and chronic obstructive pulmonary disease in stable patients, and even more so during acute exacerbations.

- Chronic nitrofurantoin induced lung disease. This lady had been on long-term nitrofurantoin and her presentation, with insidious shortness of breath over months, is in keeping with nitrofurantoin-induced lung disease. In particular she has:
  - Pulmonary infiltrates and fibrosis (right hemithorax volume loss, with tracheal deviation to the right, and reticular shadowing)
  - Eosinophilia (count 1.1×10^9/L)
  - Bronchospasm (previously diagnosed as 'late onset asthma')
  - Positive antinuclear antibody: a drug-induced lupus.

Other pulmonary complications of nitrofurantoin are listed at www.
pneumotox.com, and include;

◆ Acute nitrofurantoin-induced lung disease which usually has an abrupt
   onset within 3 weeks of starting the drug with fevers, chills, cough,
   dyspnoea, abnormal CXR, leucocytosis and eosinophilia. It usually
   resolves after the drug is discontinued.

◆ Subacute nitrofurantoin-induced lung disease, associated with an
   eosinophilia, vasculitis and hypersensitivity.

◆ Chronic nitrofurantoin-induced lung disease, which much less
   common, and is characterized by increasing dyspnoea on exertion,
   dry cough, bilateral diffuse infiltrates and fibrosis, more prominent at
   the lung bases, often with a pleural effusion.

It is not clear what phase of the disease our patient was in, as she has
features of each. The acute and chronic forms of lung injury result from
different pathogenic mechanisms. The acute form is a hypersensitivity
reaction (type I or III). The chronic form may be either an allergic or a
toxic response. Theoretically, hyperoxia accelerates toxicity, and antioxidants protect from toxicity through cyclic oxidation and reduction. This
mechanism of lung damage may be similar to that observed with the
herbicide paraquat.

Nitrofurantoin-induced lung disease is not a dose-related phenomenon,
and the incidence is higher in women, simply because they are more
prone to urinary tract infections and, therefore, receive more treatment
with nitrofurantoin. One study has found the incidence of hospitalization following a single prescription to be just under 1 in 5000, and of 742
people with >10 prescriptions of nitrofurantoin, there was one fatal case
attributable to the drug. Non-pulmonary manifestations of nitrofurantoin
include mild gastro-intestinal symptoms, acute allergic reactions, hepatic,
neurological and haematological toxicity.

◆ Amiodarone-induced lung disease. Amiodarone is one of the commonest drugs to induce lung disease, and should be considered in this
   lady's case given her history of dysrhythmias. However, review of her
   notes documented no amiodarone use.

23b) **What step is important to try and halt the progression of her underlying
   condition?**

Key management to try and halt disease progression:

◆ Nitrofurantoin must be discontinued as soon as an adverse drug reaction is suspected. Prognosis depends upon the drug reaction and how
   soon the complication is recognized and nitrofurantoin withdrawn.

Following an acute reaction, the prognosis is good. Following chronic lung disease, drug withdrawal may lead to an improvement; however, mortality is still 10%. The role of corticosteroids in nitrofurantoin-induced lung disease has not been properly evaluated.

◆ For the suspected UIP component of her disease, drug treatment is not used routinely. Oral corticosteroids alone, or in combination with azathioprine, may improve lung function and survival, though studies supporting their use probably included some patients with pulmonary fibrosis other than UIP, such as non-specific interstitial pneumonitis, which is steroid responsive.

Further progress

Intra-venous amoxicillin and oral erythromycin were given for a community acquired pneumonia. Her shortness of breath improved a little, and the CRP fell; inspiratory crackles and CXR changes persisted. A CT was performed (Fig. 23.2).

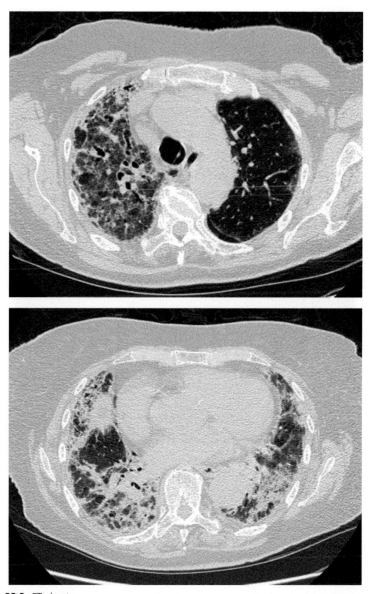

Fig. 23.2 CT chest.

Questions

23c) Describe the CT chest changes.

23d) What further investigations could be considered?

Answers

23c) **Describe the CT chest changes.**

The CT shows ground glass opacification associated with traction dilatation and bronchiectasis, and areas of coarse reticulation and honeycombing. In the upper zones on CT, changes predominate on the right. Appearances would be in keeping with severe usual interstitial pneumonitis, although the asymmetrical distribution would be unusual.

23d) **What further investigations could be considered?**

An open lung biopsy is sometimes helpful in cases of pulmonary fibrosis where there is doubt regarding the underlying diagnosis. Full pulmonary function tests aid assessment at sequential follow-up. This lady was not sufficiently stable to be considered for this.

Early recognition of drug toxicity is important as it is a common cause of morbidity and even mortality. Unfortunately the lady in this case went on to develop progressive fibrosis and secondary pulmonary infection, and died 3 months after initial presentation.

Further reading

Jick SS, Jick H, Walker AM, Hunter JR (1989). Hospitalization for pulmonary reactions following nitrofurantoin use. *Chest*; **96**: 512–515.

Martin WJ (1991). Pharmacologic and other chemical causes of interstitial lung disease. *Chest*; **100**: 231–233.

Schattner A, Von der Walde J, Kozak N, Sokolovskaya N, Knobler H (1999). Nitrofurantoin-induced immune-mediated lung and liver disease. *Am J Med Sci*; **317** (5): 336–340.

Case 24

A 45-year-old engineer (born 1943) was referred by his GP for possible sleep apnoea in 1988. His presenting complaint was increasing and severe daytime sleepiness (he had fallen asleep whilst on the telephone and driving), general tiredness and fatigue, and restless sleep. He was known to be a snorer, but not every night. He had been a smoker for 25 years, having given up recently. He had had rheumatic fever aged 6 and a squint operation aged 8. Aged 16 he was 6ft 2in but by 17 he had lost 2in and was noticed to have a scoliosis. By aged 20 this was bad enough to require a spinal fusion. On examination he was 5ft 9in and thin (BMI 21). Apart from the scoliosis there was no evidence of a neuromuscular abnormality, in particular no fasciculation; nor evidence of cor pulmonale.

Investigations

Formal sleep study (Fig. 24.3) showed that the episodes of worsening hypoxaemia were during REM sleep, and there was no evidence of obstructive sleep apnoea.

Pulmonary junction (Table 24.1) and blood gases (Table 24.2) were as follows.

Table 24.1 Pulmonary function tests

		% Predicted
PEFR(L/m)	375	75
FEV_1(L)	1.6	48
FVC(L, standing)	2.2	53
FVC(L, lying)	2.1	51
FEV_1/VC(%)	72	low normal
FRC(L)	2.3	66
RV(L)	1.4	59
TLC(L)	3.6	53
RV/TLC(%)	38	33
RAW(kPa/L/s)	0.14	(<0.2)
SGAW(L/s.kPa)	3.1	normal
TL_{CO}(mmol/min/kPa)	5.3	56
K_{CO}(mmol/min/kPa/L)	1.70	115
PiMax(cmH$_2$O)	33	low normal
PeMax(cmH$_2$O)	95	normal

Table 24.2 Blood gases

PaO_2(kPa)	6.81	SaO_2(%)	88
$PaCO_2$(kPa)	7.65	standard $[HCO_3]^-$ (mmol/l)	30.6
pH	7.34	Aa gradient (kPa)	3.6

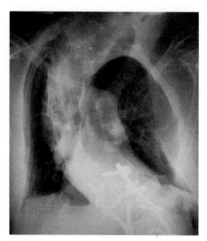

Fig. 24.1 Chest radiograph.

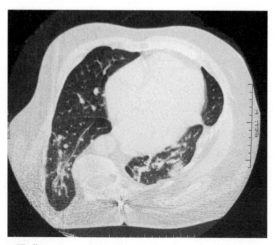

Fig. 24.2 Chest CT slice.

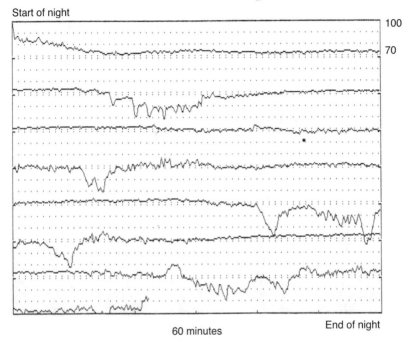

Fig. 24.3 Eight sequential hours of oximetry taken from the sleep study.

Questions

24a) What abnormalities do the lung function tests show?

24b) What abnormalities do the blood gases show?

24c) Can the lung function tests explain the blood gases?

24d) Does the CXR and CT slice help?

24e) Does the sleep study help?

24f) What general group of disorders are these abnormal findings likely to result from?

Answers

24a) **What abnormalities do the lung function tests show?**

Lung function shows a restrictive defect with no evidence of additional airways obstruction. Lung volume measurements are about 50% predicted. The FEV_1/VC ratio is slightly low; however, there is no evidence of air trapping (normal RV/TLC ratio), increased airways obstruction or decreased conductance. The K_{CO} is slightly raised, as one would expect if there was failure to expand otherwise relatively normal lung. The preserved FVC on lying down essentially rules out diaphragm weakness. The expiratory mouth pressure is well preserved; the inspiratory pressure is a little low, either due to weak muscles or mechanically disadvantaged muscles, as occurs in scoliosis.

24b) **What abnormalities do the blood gases show?**

The blood gases show a partially compensated, mild ventilatory failure with a small increase in Aa gradient.

24c) **Can the lung function tests explain the blood gases?**

Lung function and blood gases. In patients with a scoliosis, the VC usually has to fall to about a litre before ventilatory failure occurs. With neuromuscular causes of ventilatory failure, it has been shown that the lying VC is the most predictive of diurnal CO_2 retention, and usually needs to fall to below 25% predicted normal. Thus to be in ventilatory failure with a lying VC over 2L would be *very* unusual, and requires additional explanation. This might be obesity (but he is thin), additional airways obstruction (e.g. from his smoking, but the lung function does not support significant airways obstruction) or a neuromuscular cause of weakness (for which there is no obvious supporting evidence).

24d) **Does the CXR and CT slice help?**

The CXR (Fig. 24.1) shows the expected scoliosis, with the vertebral stabilisation applied to the lumbar area, rather than the thoracic. The CT slice (Fig. 24.2) shows areas of probable atelectasis from failure to adequately expand parts of the lung, the likely explanation for the raised Aa gradient.

24e) **Does the sleep study help?**

The sleep study (Fig. 24.3) shows a stable reduction in SaO_2 during non-REM sleep, and yet further large unstable falls in SaO_2 during REM sleep, but none of the recurrent saw-tooth oxygen desaturations typical of obstructive sleep apnoea. This would be typical of any ventilatory failure patient, from many different causes, e.g. neuromuscular, COPD, obesity and scoliosis, as here.

24f) **What general group of disorders are these abnormal findings likely to result from?**

The likely cause is not clear at all, and one is either looking at two unrelated diagnoses (e.g. an additional brain stem abnormality such as Arnold Chiari malformation), or a rare neurological diagnosis that could cause both a central control abnormality and the late onset scoliosis.

Questions

24g) Suggest a possible single neurological diagnosis.

24h) What additional tests might help confirm this diagnosis?

Answers

24g) **Suggest a possible single neurological diagnosis.**

Previous polio might explain the findings, but cannot be proven.

24h) **What additional tests might help confirm this diagnosis?**

Electrophysiological studies might show evidence of previous denervation and re-innervation in multiple areas of the body. They, in fact, did show evidence of motor unit action potentials increased in size and prolonged in duration, compared to normal (suggesting that surviving anterior horn cells were innervating greater numbers of muscle fibres than normal). These changes were present in several areas. There were no fibrillation potentials to imply ongoing motor axon loss. These findings were interpreted as showing widespread evidence of chronic motor neurone loss. This patient is now nearly 20 years on from the original presentation with ventilatory failure and he shows no evidence of increasing weakness.

Poliomyelitis is caused by a highly infectious enterovirus that gains entry via the GI tract, having been excreted in faeces from an active case. It reproduces in the pharynx and GI tract for 2 weeks or so, before being either contained, or producing a viraemia with signs of meningeal irritation. Even at this stage, only about two-thirds will go on to detectable paralysis. Over 90% of infections do not produce an episode of 'aseptic meningitis' or muscle weakness, but are simply diagnosed as a pharyngitis or 'flu'; evidence for this comes from epidemiological viral antibody studies. It is thought that over 50% of the anterior horn cells supplying a muscle need to be destroyed in the acute phase to produce noticeable weakness. Recovery of weakness is due to re-innervation of orphaned muscle fibres. Scoliosis can develop after the original involvement of the paravertebral muscles (due to unbalanced spinal support with bending away from the weaker affected side), usually during a subsequent growth spurt some while later. Electrophysiological studies show that many muscle groups, not originally thought to have been involved, show evidence of chronic denervation, indicating more widespread 'involvement' than symptomatically evident. In addition to involvement of anterior horn cells supplying peripheral muscles, there is clinical and post-mortem evidence of neuronal damage in other areas. For example, there is a bulbar form that can involve the brainstem areas controlling autonomic function, pharyngeal function and ventilatory control. Such cases tended to be severe and patients rarely survive without ventilatory

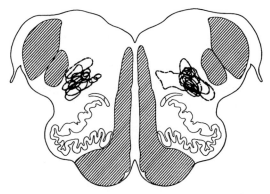

Fig. 24.4 Superimposed medullary lesions (dashed black lines) from 17 patients who died of ventilatory failure secondary to bulbar poliomyelitis. Located in the lateral reticular formation. From Baker *et al.* (1950). *Arch Neurol Psychiat*; 63: 257–281.

support. Figure 24.4 shows the areas in the brainstem that need to be destroyed by poliovirus to produce acute ventilatory failure.

Many years after the original polio (usually 20–40 years later), there can be an increase or return of weakness in areas previously affected; this has been termed 'post-polio syndrome'. The mechanism of this is not clear. Suggestions that it is due to persisting virus and new anterior horn cell damage, have no real supporting evidence. Joints that suffered from loss of some muscle support, and thus mechanical imbalance, can be gradually damaged over time, with the resulting osteoarthritis producing new disability. The favoured explanation is that the surviving anterior horn cells originally sprouted new branches to re-innervate the orphaned muscle fibres and that, after many years, they prematurely age due to the 'over-use' of having to supply more muscle fibres. There is evidence of increased fatigability of muscles from polio survivors, which may explain the complaint of excess fatigue typical of this syndrome. In addition, there can be apparently inexplicable problems, such as dysphagia, autonomic dysfunction and ventilatory failure. The predictors of late ventilatory failure are respiratory muscle involvement (with a period on a ventilator) during the original polio, and the presence of significant scoliosis. Further subsequent decline is usually very slow. Modafinil does not help the fatigue. There is early evidence that intravenous immunoglobulin may improve symptoms; if true, then there may be alternative explanations for the syndrome, besides those suggested above.

To diagnose post-polio syndrome requires (Farbu *et al.* 2006):

- A history of paralytic polio; confirmed or not confirmed; partial or fairly complete initial recovery.
- After a period of functional stability of at least 15 years, development of new muscle dysfunction: muscle weakness, muscle atrophy, muscle pain and fatigue.
- Neurological examination compatible with prior polio: lower motor neurone lesions; decreased or absent tendon reflexes; no sensory loss; compatible findings on EMG and/or MRI.

Thus this patient does *not* have the full house to allow a diagnosis of post-polio syndrome; the vast majority of such patients do have a clear history of previous polio. However, it is possible that he contracted apparently asymptomatic polio in his early teens (during the polio epidemics of the 1950s), which involved his thoracic paravertebral muscles, mainly on the right, and perhaps with partial bulbar damage as well. During his adolescent growth spurt a scoliosis subsequently developed. Some 35 years later, the combination of the scoliosis and possible partial bulbar damage led to mild ventilatory failure with marked nocturnal hypoventilation, particularly during REM sleep when compensatory ventilatory mechanisms are least effective due to the muscle paralysis accompanying normal REM sleep.

Progress

This patient was placed on non-invasive ventilation overnight with normalization of both his sleep study (Fig. 24.5) and $PaCO_2$ (PaO_2 9.7, $PaCO_2$ 5.6, base excess −1.5). He has remained well for nearly 20 years and his FVC is stable at 2L; this would further support a diagnosis of post-polio effects, rather than any alternative progressive neuro-muscular disorder. If he tries not to use his ventilator at night, his sleep is again disrupted, and by the fourth night his $PaCO_2$ is again abnormally raised.

Eight sequential hours of oximetry –
each line 70–100% SaO$_2$

Start of night

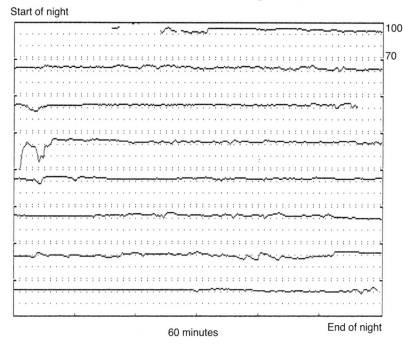

60 minutes   End of night

Fig. 24.5 Eight sequential hours of oximetry taken from the sleep study.

Further reading

Bach JR (1995). Management of post-polio respiratory sequelae. *Ann N Y Acad Sci*; **753**: 96–102.

Farbu E, Gilhus NE, Barnes MP, Borg K, deVisser M, Driessen A *et al.* (2006). EFNS guideline on diagnosis and management of post-polio syndrome. *European Journal of Neurology*; **13**: 795–801.

Howard RS (2005). Poliomyelitis and the postpolio syndrome. *BMJ*; **330**: 1314–1318.

Case 25

A 40-year-old woman presented to A&E with pleuritic right-sided chest pain. This had occurred suddenly whilst at rest, and was associated with shallow breathing. She had a past history of dysmenorrhoea, investigated with a laparoscopy with no positive findings two years previously, but was otherwise fit and well. She was currently on day three of her period. She was a lifelong non-smoker, with two healthy children. On examination, she was tachypnoeic (20/min) with oxygen saturations of 96% on air, and decreased breath sounds on the right side. Her CXR is shown in Fig. 25.1.

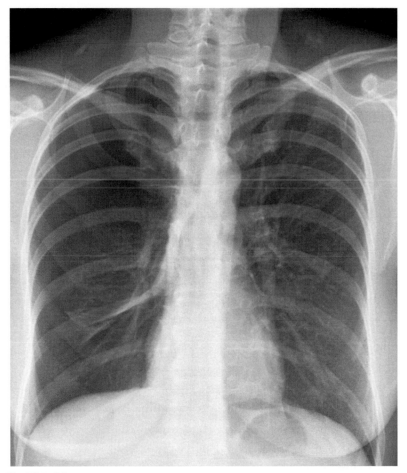

Fig. 25.1 CXR.

Questions

25a) What is the diagnosis?

25b) How would you quantify its size?

25c) What is the relevance of size to treatment?

25d) How would you treat this patient and why?

25e) What is the prognosis from this condition?

25f) What counselling does she require on discharge?

Answers

25a) **What is the diagnosis?**

The diagnosis at this stage is of primary, spontaneous pneumothorax (PSP). Although the history of previous dysmenorhoea is of interest, after a first episode of pneumothorax a diagnosis of catamenial pneumothorax (related to the menstrual cycle) cannot be made confidently. This diagnosis requires recurrent pneumothoraces within 72h before or after the onset of menstruation. The presence of endothoracic endometrial tissue is not required for a diagnosis.

25b) **How would you quantify its size?**

There are several ways in which to score the size of a pneumothorax, recommended in management guidelines. All take into account that estimation of a volume change on a two-dimensional image (i.e. the CXR) is inaccurate. Some authors have suggested a simple classification scoring pneumothorax into 'large' (complete dehiscence of the lung from the chest wall, as seen here, Fig. 25.2) and 'small or moderate' (partial dehiscence). American and British guidelines (see reading list) recommend different cut-offs for size of pneumothorax: >2cm rim large (UK) or >3cm rim large (USA). While there are complex research tools available to calculate the degree of lung collapse, a reasonable clinical tool is the 'Light index'. This approximates pneumothorax size using the cube of the lung diameter to hemithorax diameter (see Fig. 25.2).

25c) **What is the relevance of size to treatment?**

Aetiology and clinical status of the patient determines which treatment strategy to use, rather than precise calculations of pneumothorax volume.

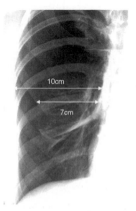

(Hemithorax d^3 – lung d^3) / Hemithorax d^3

$(10^3 - 7^3) / 10^3 = $ **66% pneumothorax**

10cm

7cm

Fig. 25.2 CXR showing calculation of the Light index, which has been shown to closely correlate with the amount of air obtained at aspiration.

This is especially important in patients with secondary pneumothorax (i.e. in the presence of underlying lung disease), where the lung may not collapse due to air trapping in the underlying lung, or be tethered, giving the appearance of a small pneumothorax on PA CXR. In secondary pneumothorax, even small pneumothoraces can cause significant symptoms and 'tension'. Intervention is recommended in patients with 'large' pneumothoraces in guidelines, but the clinical state of the patient should be the first assessment tool and trump the guidelines. In the presence of complete pneumothorax (total lung collapse), aspiration or drainage is likely to be required due to symptoms and the theoretical risk of tensioning.

25d) How would you treat this patient and why?

Possible treatment strategies in first episode of PSP are shown in Table 25.1.

If sufficiently symptomatic, the likely best treatment strategy in this case is aspiration (on the basis of no difference in outcomes listed in Table 25.1 and potentially decreased risks). There is a large pneumothorax on radiology in association with symptoms, requiring intervention, with a high possible success rate from aspiration, which may avoid the need for admission. Drain placement is associated with significant potential risks and should be considered carefully before being used as a treatment for this disease.

25e) What is the prognosis from this condition?

As above, the prognosis of PSP is good, and it should be regarded as an inconvenient but benign disease (mortality 0.09% in men, 0.06% in women). This is in contrast to secondary pneumothorax (in the presence of underlying lung disease) which is associated with a 10–15% mortality. Recurrence rates after a first episode PSP are between 16 and 57%, with a mean of 30%, and most occur within 2 years of initial event. Smoking cessation is a key component to management, as recurrence is up to 9 times more likely in continuing smokers.

25f) What counselling does she require on discharge?

Post-PSP resolution, patients should be advised to stop smoking, if relevant, and advised about flying and diving. Patients who have experienced even a single PSP may not dive with pressurized breathing equipment (snorkling is considered safe) unless a surgical pleurodesis has been conducted. Previous guidelines suggested patients should wait for at least 6 weeks before flying after radiological resolution has occurred, but more recent guidelines suggest that patients may safely fly after 1 week of radiological resolution. Patients with active pneumothoraces may not fly (pneumothorax air expansion causing respiratory compromise at lower

Table 25.1 Pneumothorax management

Management	Evidence
Conservative (no intervention, early follow up with CXR)	PSP is a benign disease with <0.1% mortality or tension. Spontaneous resolution of pneumothorax volume occurs at 1–2% of hemithorax volume per day. Must ensure no evidence of progression (i.e. no ongoing air leak).
Aspiration (Aspiration may be conducted using an intravenous cannula system or specially designed catheter aspiration kits. These kits consist of an 8F catheter passed in to the chest over a guide-wire with a 3-way tap. The success of initial aspiration may be checked with radiology without removing the catheter, and re-aspiration conducted, if required.)	Aspiration successful in 59–73% of PSP in five randomized trials comparing aspiration to intercostal drainage. Cochrane review of trials (including only one study) showed no difference between drainage and aspiration in: • Immediate success rate • Early (1-month) failure rate • Duration of hospital stay • Need for pleurodesis at 1 year • Decreased number of admissions with aspiration. Pilot studies suggest good success rates from aspiration kits. In PSP, increased size of pneumothorax is associated with increased likelihood of treatment failure.
Intercostal Drainage	Good success rates and permits assessment of ongoing air leak (drain can be left in for several days). Requires admission and associated with an up to 5% infection (empyema) rate. Pleurodesis may be conducted through an intercostal drain on resolution of pneumothorax, but this is not recommended in PSP (although widely practised in Europe).
Thoracic Surgery	Highly successful in treatment and prevention (around 95% for thoracotomy, somewhat lower for mini-thoracotomy and video-assisted thoracoscopic surgery (VATs)). Two studies demonstrating cost saving using VATs as initial treatment for first episode and recurrent pneumothorax. Mean recurrence rate in PSP after one episode is 30%; therefore, 70% of patients will not require further treatment after the 1st episode. Surgery therefore not recommended after first episode.

pressures). Once full resolution has occurred clinically and radiologically, the theoretical risk of flying is of a recurrence occurring at altitude. As this may occur in 30% of patients (i.e. the minority) over a 2-year period, a pragmatic approach has now been taken.

Progress

The patient was successfully treated with a single aspiration, with good radiological result. She was counselled and discharged and at follow-up 1 month later was well, although remained anxious about possible recurrence.

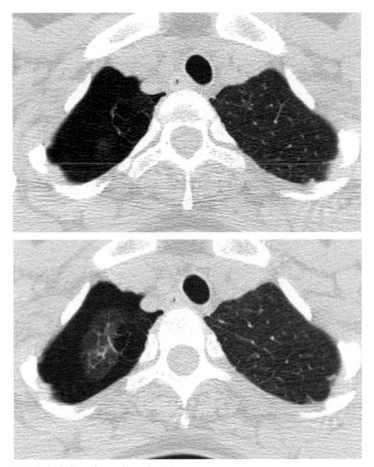

Fig. 25.3 Apical slices from thoracic CT.

She represented 4 months later with the same symptoms (not during menstruation), and was found to have a moderate right pneumothorax. She refused further aspiration or chest drain insertion, and requested surgical intervention. A CT (Fig. 25.3) scan was therefore performed.

Questions

25g) What does the CT show (Fig. 25.3)?

25h) Does the CT inform aetiology or treatment options?

25i) What are the surgical options available?

Answers

25g) **What does the CT show (Fig. 25.3)?**

The CT (Fig. 25.3) shows a current right-sided pneumothorax and small subpleural blebs and bullae (arrows) collectively known as emphysema-like changes (ELCs) (Fig. 25.4).

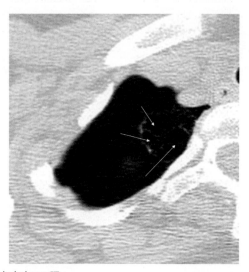

Fig. 25.4 Expanded chest CT.

25h) **Does the CT inform aetiology or treatment options?**

Treatment options. After a second PSP, recurrence rates are higher (around 50%) and decisions of medical management versus surgical treatment are largely dependent on patient choice. In the case of a third episode ipsilaterally, ongoing air leak or first evidence of bilateral pneumothorax (usually on separate occasions), surgical intervention is recommended. The decision to operate is not usually based on CT appearances.

Aetiology of PSP. The aetiology of PSP is unknown. ELCs may be the areas of parenchymal air leak in PSP, and are found in 90% of cases at thoracotomy and 80% of cases using HRCT in both smokers and non-smokers with PSP, in comparison to 25% of matched controls without PSP. PSP patients are taller than average, and it is postulated that the increased gradient in pleural pressure may lead to bleb and bulla formation and result in PSP. However, ELCs have not been convincingly shown to predict first or recurrent pneumothorax.

Direct evidence from thoracotomy suggests that observed air leak from ELCs is highly variable (between 4 and 75% of cases). Studies have demonstrated that recurrence rate is higher in patients treated with bullectomy alone compared to bullectomy plus pleurodesis, arguing against all PSP being a result of ELC leakage. Interesting data, using inhaled fluoroscein to assess the site of air leak at thoracoscopy, suggest that areas not associated with visible bullae are often responsible. Resected specimens from pneumothorax lungs demonstrate small airways inflammation almost universally, suggesting that the pathology may be more widespread within the lung parenchyma.

The CT appearances, therefore, do not change the treatment options in this case, although most thoracic surgeons would conduct a pleurodesis and blebectomy in this situation. Further studies are required to assess the validity of this approach.

25i) **What are the surgical options available?**

Surgical options:

♦ Open thoracotomy—demonstrates the best results, usually pleurectomy performed during the procedure. A pneumothorax recurrence rate of around 1% is quoted. However, chronic post-thoracotomy pain is common, occurring in 75% of patients at 6 months and 61% one year after surgery.

♦ Mini-thoracotomy—less invasive than above (5cm axillary scar) and a recurrence rate comparable to open thoracotomy is reported.

♦ Video-assisted thoracoscopic surgery—even less invasive but with a reported recurrence rate of 5–10%.

Further reading

Baumann MH, Noppen M (2004). Pneumothorax. *Respirology*; **9**: 157–164.

Baumann MH, Strange C, Heffner JE *et al.* (2001). Management of spontaneous pneumothorax: an American College of Chest Physicians Delphi consensus statement. *Chest*; **119**: 590–602.

Henry M, Arnold T, Harvey J (2003). BTS guidelines for the management of spontaneous pneumothorax. *Thorax*; **58** Suppl 2: ii39–ii52.

Case 26

A 70-year-old man was admitted with severe dyspnoea, paroxysmal nocturnal dyspnoea and an unproductive cough that had progressed over 4 days. He gave a background history of minor exertional breathlessness over the last 6 months. A CXR 3 months previously had raised concern over a pulmonary nodule, and this had prompted a CT confirming multiple subpleural nodules, up to 16mm in size, along with borderline enlargement of mediastinal and axillary lymph nodes. An interval CT to assess any change was awaited at the time of his acute presentation. His background was of Type II diabetes mellitus (15 years duration), hypertension and mild chronic renal failure (recent urea 8.0mmol/L, and creatinine 151μmol/L). Systemic enquiry revealed intermittent nasal blockage, discharge and crusting. On examination he had a sinus tachycardia of 115, respiratory rate of 25/min, SaO_2 of 26% on FiO_2 0.6 and BP 105/70. JVP was not seen and there was peripheral oedema to both knees. Heart sounds were normal, and chest examination revealed reduced air entry at both bases and fine crackles to both upper zones.

Investigations

- Arterial blood gas (on 60% O_2): PaO_2 9.7kPa, $PaCO_2$ 4.5kPa, pH 7.42, $[HCO_3]^-$ 26 mmol/L
- Urinalysis, + protein, trace non-haemolysed blood
- Urea 16.2mmol/L, creatinine 202μmol/L, LFT normal, CRP 64mg/L, ESR 37mm/h
- Hb 8.4g/dL (previous Hb 8.9), MCV 85fl, WCC 11.3×10^9/L (eosinophils 0.45×10^9/L), Plts 445×10^9/L
- Serum ferritin 201.8ng/mL (20–300), iron 15.0μmol/L (14–31), transferrin 1.97g/L (1.8–3.6), B12/folate normal; blood film showed normochromic, normocytic red cells.

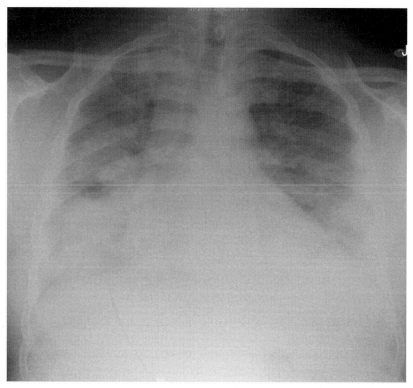

Fig. 26.1 CXR.

Questions

26a) Interpret the CXR (Fig. 26.1).

26b) What is the most likely diagnosis and underlying cause for his acute presentation?

26c) What other diagnoses should be considered?

26d) What further investigation should be done?

Answers

26a) **Interpret the CXR (Fig. 26.1).**

The CXR (Fig. 26.1) shows that the heart is enlarged. There is bilateral perihilar and lower zone consolidation with airspace opacification extending to the apices. There are bilateral effusions.

26b) **What is the most likely diagnosis and underlying cause for his acute presentation?**

The most likely diagnosis is acute pulmonary oedema, although the CXR is not entirely typical. With his risk-factor profile, coronary artery disease would be the most likely underlying cause for this. Additional issues that require explanation are the deteriorating renal function and anaemia. A possible cause for this would be progressive diabetic nephropathy with an anaemia of chronic disease. It would, however, be unusual for erythropoietin deficiency to cause anaemia at this level of renal dysfunction, and iron studies are difficult to interpret in acute illness.

26c) **What other diagnoses should be considered?**

Other causes of diffuse pulmonary infiltrates should be considered such as infection, adult respiratory distress syndrome (ARDS), other inflammatory processes (e.g. organizing pneumonia, acute interstitial pneumonitis), vasculitis or pulmonary haemorrhage.

26d) **What further investigation should be done?**

Further investigations would include:

- Cardiac troponin and echo
- Blood and urine cultures
- Spot urine protein/creatinine ratio (PCR)
- Urine microscopy for casts
- ANCA
- Renal ultrasound
- Consider CT chest and pulmonary function tests, if no improvement with initial therapy.

Progress

Further investigations

- Cardiac troponin negative.
- Echo showed normal left and right ventricular systolic function and no valvular abnormalities. There was no suggestion of diastolic dysfunction, nor evidence of pulmonary hypertension.

- Urine protein/creatinine ratio 120mg/mmol (levels over 300mg/mmol generally considered nephrotic).
- Urine microscopy negative for red cell casts.
- c-ANCA positive at 1/40 titre, anti-PR3 43.7U/mL(0–6), anti-MPO 21.1U/mL(0–6).
- Renal ultrasound normal.

Following an initial bolus of 50mg furosemide and 2 days treatment with 40mg furosemide once daily, the patient remained dyspnoeic and hypoxic with no improvement in his CXR appearances. Haemoglobin levels did not change significantly and there was no growth on urine or blood cultures. The patient was too unwell to perform reliable pulmonary function tests. A CT scan was performed (Fig. 26.2).

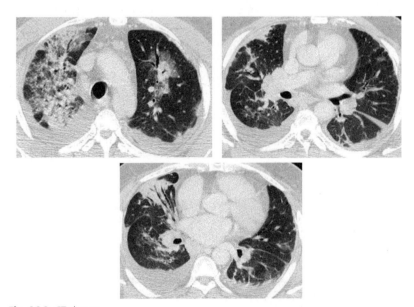

Fig. 26.2 CT thorax.

Questions

26e) Interpret the CT scan (Fig. 26.2).

26f) What diagnosis are the appearances most consistent with?

Answers

26e) **Interpret the CT scan (Fig. 26.2).**

The CT (Fig. 26.2) shows an enlarged heart, bilateral pleural effusions, bilateral ground glass opacification in a predominantly central and upper zone distribution. There are areas of peripheral consolidation. There is also interlobar septal thickening (Fig. 26.3), which is not irregular or nodular. The lymphadenopathy identified on the initial CT (not shown) had not changed significantly but the parenchymal changes were obscuring the previously identified nodules and so it was not possible to comment on any interval changes to them.

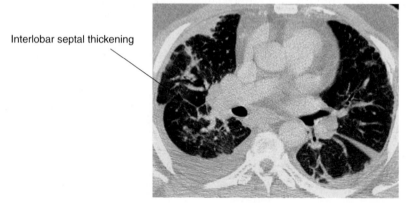

Interlobar septal thickening

Fig. 26.3 Selected CT section.

Interlobar septal thickening is commonly caused by fluid, where the thickening is smooth, or malignant infiltration of lymphatics (lymphangitis), where it is more nodular. It can also be a finding in interstitial fibrosis (irregular septal thickening) and rarely in bronchiectasis.

26f) **What diagnosis are the appearances most consistent with?**

Despite the previously normal echo, these appearances are most consistent with ongoing pulmonary oedema. The positive ANCA raised concerns of vasculitis, and hence pulmonary haemorrhage should be considered. The CT appearances are not those of vasculitis or pulmonary haemorrhage, and the lack of any change in haemoglobin would also go against pulmonary haemorrhage.

There is often wide inter-observer variation in the reporting of left ventricular systolic function (LVSF) on USS, but even if LVSF appears normal, diastolic dysfunction (especially in hypertensive patients) alone can cause clinically evident heart failure.

Progress

More aggressive diuretic treatment was commenced, which did improve the situation symptomatically and radiologically. A repeat cardiac USS was performed, which was again reported as normal. Subsequently, renal artery stenosis (unilateral, left-sided) was demonstrated by MR angiography. The renal team advised that this would not have been a cause for his pulmonary oedema, as it was unilateral and not an especially tight stenosis; therefore, no further intervention for this was recommended. In addition, a myocardial perfusion scan showed no evidence of regional ischaemia. The precise cause of his pulmonary oedema remained unclear and the cardiologists did not recommend coronary angiography. Repeat C-ANCA titre remained 1/40 with Anti-PR3 of 123U/mL and creatinine remained around 200µmol/L.

The renal team suggested that diabetic nephropathy, and not renal vasculitis, was responsible for the chronic renal impairment. A renal biopsy was not felt to be necessary at this point.

At chest clinic review 2 months later he had a residual cough and reduced exercise tolerance with dyspnoea at 200 yards. Clinical examination revealed no evidence of cardiac decompensation and a clear chest.

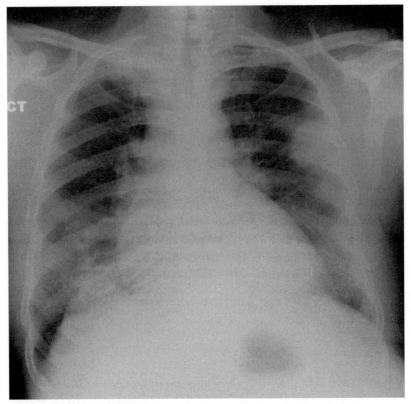

Fig. 26.4 CXR at chest clinic review.

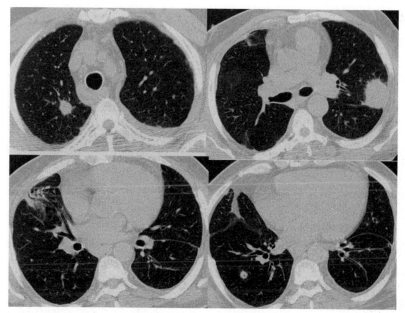

Fig. 26.5 Interval CT thorax.

Questions

26g) Interpret the CXR (Fig. 26.4) and CT (Fig. 26.5).

26h) What is the next investigation?

Answers

26g) **Interpret the CXR (Fig. 26.4) and CT (Fig. 26.5).**

The most striking abnormality shown on the CXR (Fig. 26.4) and the CT (Fig. 26.5) is the development of a fairly rounded opacity in the left-upper zone, which may be pleurally based. There is also some persisting atelectasis in the right-lower zone. Although the heart appears enlarged, there does not appear to be any persisting pulmonary oedema.

The CT (Fig. 26.5) also shows bilateral spiculated nodules of varying size, with evidence of cavitation in the right-lower lobe nodule. In addition, there is an area of consolidation anteriorly in the RLL. There is right paratracheal lymphadenopathy.

26h) **What is the next investigation?**

Core biopsy of left-upper lobe lesion would be the best next investigation, although a nasal mucosal biopsy might have helped.

The differential diagnosis is of Wegener's granulomatosis, organizing pneumonia and multi-focal intra-thoracic malignancy (including lymphoma). Eosinophilc pneumonia should be considered, but would be discounted by lack of peripheral eosinophilia. Core biopsy of the lung lesion is, therefore, required to differentiate these. Although the right paratracheal node would be amenable to tansbronchial needle aspiration, the only diagnosis this could realistically secure would be of carcinoma.

Core biopsy was performed. Tissue obtained showed patchy chronic inflammation including epithelioid macrophages. No well formed granulomas were seen nor tissue necrosis. No vasculitis was observed.

Questions

26i) What final investigation is required?

26j) What is your diagnosis?

26k) What drug treatment would you commence?

Answers

26i) **What final investigation is required?**

Renal biopsy. This is required to determine therapeutic strategy (see below). Histology of this showed no evidence of renal vasculitis, but established diabetic nephropathy only.

26j) **What is your diagnosis?**

Non-renal Wegener's granulomatosis. Despite the lung biopsy not confirming pathologically evident vasculitis, results so far are in keeping with a systemic vasculitis involving the upper (nasal symptoms initially described) and lower respiratory tract.

26k) **What drug treatment would you commence?**

The management will be in two phases, namely induction and maintenance of remission. Previous conventional treatment of ANCA-associated systemic vasculitis would be combined cyclophosphamide and high-dose prednisolone for induction, with cyclophosphamide continued for at least one year and prednisolone gradually tapered over this time. This leads to remission in about 90% of cases. Concern regarding toxicity of cyclophosphamide (bone-marrow toxicity, infection, myeloproliferative diseases) has led to recent studies addressing alternative, potentially less toxic treatment regimens.

Recent evidence has suggested that in patients with systemic ANCA-associated vasculitis (Wegener's or microscopic polyangiitis), but without life-threatening features (including severe haemoptysis with bilateral infiltrates) or significantly impaired renal function (creatinine >150µmol/L), induction of remission can just as effectively be achieved with methotrexate (MTX) as with cyclophosphamide (CYC) (de Groot *et al.* 2005). In this study, patients received either 15mg/week MTX ($n = 49$) increasing to maximum 20–25mg/week by 12 weeks for a total of 12 months, or 2mg/kg/day CYC ($n = 46$) for 3–6 months. At remission, CYC was reduced to 1.5mg/kg/day until month 10, when it was tapered and stopped by 12 months. Both groups received prednisolone 1mg/kg/day for 12 weeks, then tapered to 15mg/day at 12 weeks, 7.5mg/day at 6 months and stopped at 12 months. Most (89) had Wegener's and about half in each arm had lung involvement. At 6 months, the remission rate in the MTX group (44/49, 89.8%) was not statistically significantly less than the rate in the CYC group (43/46, 93.5%). Time to remission with MTX was longer in the subgroup with respiratory tract involvement (nodules and/or cavities and/or pulmonary infiltrates). Relapse rates at

18 months of 69.5 and 46.5% in MTX and CYC groups, respectively, suggests treatment should be continued beyond 12 months.

A further study (Jayne *et al.* 2003) comparing maintenance therapy with azathioprine (*n* =76), versus cyclophosphamide (*n* =79), following induction with prednisolone and cyclophosphamide, found no significant difference in relapse rates between the two treatment arms. This study included patients with life-threatening features at presentation, and approximately half in each arm had lung involvement. There are no studies comparing induction and/or maintenance regimens specifically in patients with lung involvement by systemic vasculitis.

The majority (75–90%) of patients with active Wegener's granulomatosis have p-ANCA/PR3-ANCA, and around 20% have p-ANCA/MPO-ANCA. The specificity of ANCA testing for Wegener's depends on laboratory methods used, and reaches 99% if target-antigen-specific test methods are used in combination with immunofluoresence.

Further reading

De Groot K, Rasmussen N, Bacon PA, Tervaert JW, Feighery C, Gregorini G *et al.* (2005). Randomised trial of cyclophosphamide versus methotrexate for induction of remission in early systemic antineutrophil cytoplasmic antibody associated vasculitis. *Arthritis and Rheumatism*; **52** (8): 2461–4269.

Jayne D, Rasmussen N, Andrassy K, Bacon P, Tervaert JW, Dadoniené J, *et al.* (2003). A randomised trial of maintenance therapy for vasulitis associated with antineutrophil cytoplasmic antibodies. *NEJM*; **349**: 36–44.

Langford CA, Specks U (2003). Wegener's granulomatosis and other vasculitides. In Gibson GJ, Geddes DM, Costabel U *et al.* (eds) *Respiratory Medicine* (3rd edn). Saunders, London, chapter 57.

Case 27

Three case histories are described in brief below.

Case A

A 60-year-old man with known sero-positive rheumatoid arthritis, controlled with weekly methotrexate and non-steroidal anti-inflammatory medication, presented with a left-sided pleural effusion discovered incidentally on a CXR prior to an inguinal hernia repair. He had no respiratory symptoms. Thoracic CT confirmed presence of a pleural effusion but no other abnormality, with normal appearing pleural surfaces. Pleural aspiration yielded slightly cloudy fluid, analysis of which is documented in Table 27.1 and illustrated in Fig. 27.1.

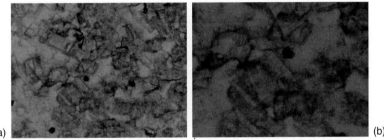

(a)   (b)

Fig. 27.1 (a) Giemsa staining and (b) birefringence of pleural fluid from patient A, demonstrating birefringent rhomboidal cholesterol crystals (courtesy of Dr Colin Clelland).

Case B

A 34-year-old woman developed sudden onset of left-sided posterior pleuritic chest pain and dyspnoea whilst stretching during yoga exercises; she was unable to continue due to pain. On examination, she was well but in obvious discomfort and had reduced air entry at her left lung base. A CXR showed small bilateral pleural effusions. These were confirmed on a CT chest, and CT pulmonary angiogram, which demonstrated no thrombo-embolic disease, lymphadenopathy or pleural abnormality. Left pleural aspiration yielded milky-coloured fluid (Fig. 27.2). Results of pleural fluid analysis are shown in Table 27.1. Her pain eased spontaneously within 24h and on review at 6 months she remained well.

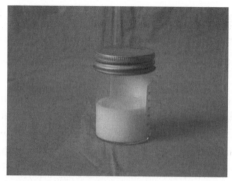

Fig. 27.2 Aspirated pleural fluid from patient B.

Case C

A 76-year-old ex-smoker (40-pack years) presented with 3 months of progressive exertional dyspnoea, anorexia with two-stone weight loss and right-sided sub-scapular pain. A CXR confirmed examination findings of a moderate pleural effusion. Pleural aspiration revealed cloudy blood-stained fluid (pleural fluid results in Table 27.1) and subsequent CT imaging showed extensive lymphadenopathy (supra-clavicular, mediastinal, paratracheal, axillary, retro-peritoneal and mesenteric) and a moderate pleural effusion with minimal pleural enhancement.

Investigations

Table 27.1 Pleural fluid results

	Patient A	Patient B	Patient C
Protein (>35g/L represents an exudate, and <25g/L a transudate)	50	41	42
Lactate dehydrogenase, (normal range 110–250IU/L)	1694	156	151
Glucose (mmol/L)	1.0	6.4	6.9
Cholesterol (mmol/L)	5.7	6.7	3.1
Triglyceride (mmol/L)	0.15	32.3	10.78
Chylomicrons	Absent	Present	Present
Cholesterol crystals	Present (see Fig. 27.1)	Absent	Absent

Questions

27a) What is the diagnosis, based on the pleural fluid analysis in each case?

27b) How could the pleural fluid aid differentiation between these diagnoses and empyema?

27c) What two conditions are commonly associated with the diagnosis in patient A? What is the prognosis?

27d) How would you investigate patient A to confirm your diagnosis?

Answers

27a) **What is the diagnosis, based on the pleural fluid analysis in each case?**
The pleural fluid analyses confirm patient A has a pseudochylothorax.

Detection of cholesterol crystals is diagnostic of a pseudochylothorax (chyliform effusion or 'cholesterol pleurisy'). However, their absence does not exclude the diagnosis. A pleural fluid cholesterol level >5.2 mmol/L (200mg/dL) is usually seen, chylomicrons are always absent.

Pseudochylothorax usually arises from a long-standing (≥5 years) pleural effusion. It is likely that lysis of cells within the pleural space releases cholesterol and lecithin–globulin complexes, which are poorly absorbed across the thickened pleural membrane.

Patients B and C each have a true chylothorax.

Diagnosis of a true chylothorax requires the presence of chylomicrons on lipoprotein electrophoresis, or a triglyceride concentration >1.24mmol/L (110mg/dL).

A chylothorax develops when there is disruption of the thoracic duct, or one of its tributaries, resulting in passage of chyle (lymph rich in chylomicrons, the macromolecules that transport fat from the intestine to the liver and adipose tissue) into the pleural space.

- The thoracic duct originates anterior to the L2 vertebra and enters the posterior mediastinum through the aortic hiatus of the diaphragm. It ascends through the thorax roughly in the mid-line, between the descending aorta on the left and the azygos vein on the right, until the level of the T5 vertebra. It then crosses to the left behind the oesophagus and continues upwards between the left side of the oesophagus and the left pleura, in the left posterior mediastinum, to above the 1st rib. After exiting the thorax it forms an arch at the level of vertebra C7, behind the jugular vein, and turns laterally and downward to empty into the venous circulation at the angle of the junction of the left jugular and subclavian veins.

- Significant anatomical variations exist.

- Injury or obstruction below where the duct traverses vertebra T5 usually results in a right-sided chylothorax, whereas disease above this point lead to a left-sided chylothorax. Cervical thoracic duct rupture may result in bilateral chylothoraces.

27b) **How could the pleural fluid aid differentiation between these diagnoses and empyema?**

The supernatant of pleural fluid from a chylothorax typically fails to clear after centrifugation, unlike with an empyema when sediment collects leaving a clear supernatant.

27c) **What two conditions are commonly associated with the diagnosis in patient A? What is the prognosis?**

The most common causes of pseudochylothoraces are: (1) tuberculous pleurisy and (2) rheumatoid pleuritis. Trauma, lung cancer, pleuropulmonary paragonimiasis and hepato-pulmonary echinococcosis may rarely cause pseudochylothoraces.

The prognosis of pseudochylothorax is usually good, although clearly depends on the underlying cause. Therapeutic thoracentesis may relieve dyspnoea but pleural fibrosis may limit symptomatic improvement and, in a minority of patients, decortication is considered. Respiratory insufficiency, pleural infection and fistulae (bronchopleural or pleurocutaneous) are rare complications.

27d) **How would you investigate patient A to confirm your diagnosis?**

Ziehl–Nielsen staining of pleural fluid and culture for acid-fast bacilli should be requested and pleural biopsies considered to exclude caseating granulomatous infiltrate. A negative interferon gamma release assay (e.g. Elispot) would effectively exclude underlying tuberculosis making it safe to assume this case is due to rheumatoid arthritis.

Questions

27e) What are the likely underlying causes in patients B and C? What is their prognosis?

27f) What other underlying conditions are associated with this diagnosis?

27g) What treatments should be considered for each patient?

Answers

27e) **What are the likely underlying causes in patients B and C? What is their prognosis?**

Patient B. Thoracic duct rupture has been described related to physical stretching and movement, which is a possible cause of the bilateral chylothoraces in this case. Formation of a localized chyle collection ('chyloma') reflects initial duct leakage and can precipitate acute chest pain and dyspnoea.

'Spontaneous' bilateral chylothoraces have been described for which no underlying cause is identified.

Patient C. The CT appearances suggested thoracic duct obstruction by malignant external lymph node compression, the most common cause for which is lymphoma. Subsequent axillary lymph node biopsy demonstrated infiltration with neoplastic follicles consistent with underlying follicular cell lymphoma.

The prognosis of chylothorax varies dependent on the underlying cause. Malignant chylothorax, chronic debilitating chylothoraces and bilateral disease carry a worse prognosis. Prompt intervention to minimize chyle loss and maximize nutritional support have improved outcome.

27f) **What other underlying conditions are associated with this diagnosis?**

Causes of true chylothorax may be classified as:

- Traumatic. Thoracic duct trauma accounts for approximately 50% of cases. Iatrogenic cases frequently arise secondary to damage during cardiothoracic surgery, i.e. aortic coarctation repair or oesophagectomy, and are a significant cause of post-operative morbidity and mortality. Other iatrogenic causes, such as central venous catheterization or pacemaker insertion, are occasionally implicated. Non-iatrogenic traumatic precipitants include blunt chest trauma (e.g. seat-belt injuries) or penetrating injury.

- Malignant. Malignancy, particularly lymphoma (70% of malignant cases), can cause thoracic duct disruption.

- Congenital. Congenital chylothorax arises from thoracic duct malformation or atresia. Birth trauma and repair of diaphragmatic defects may precipitate a chylothorax.

- Miscellaneous. Lymphangioleiomyomatosis (LAM) (see case 9) is a rare cause; in one series, 10% of patients with LAM had a chylothorax over a 25-year period.

Idiopathic chylothoraces occur in 6–15%. Spontaneous bilateral chylothoraces have been described.

27g) **What treatments should be considered for each patient?**

Patient A. As the patient is asymptomatic, if TB is excluded, no treatment is required.

Patient B. Traumatic rupture of the thoracic duct often heals spontaneously. Given patient B's clinical improvement and lack of symptoms no intervention is required.

Patient C. Treatment of malignant chylothorax should be directed at the underlying primary cancer. Resolution of the chylothorax occurs in almost 70% of patients with lymphoma following radiotherapy and chemotherapy. This patient should be referred to the haem-oncology team for appropriate management of her lymphoma.

Persistent symptoms, despite systemic therapy, warrant specific treatment of the effusion with pleural drainage, and talc pleurodesis if full lung re-expansion occurs. Pleuro-peritoneal or pleuro-venous shunting has been used in patients with no chyloascites and recycles the nutritional component of the extravasated chyle.

Management decisions for patients with chylothorax depend upon the aetiology with no randomized trial data existing to guide therapy. The universal approach should aim to: (i) optimize nutrition, (ii) relieve symptoms and (iii) close the thoracic duct defect. Identification of the leakage point during operative repair is achieved by giving the patient either a lipophilic dye or high fat content fluid, e.g. cream, orally beforehand.

♦ Post-operative chylothoraces are associated with a mortality of approximately 50%. A conservative approach with chest tube drainage and TPN may work, especially in those patients with low initial rates of fluid drainage. Immunocompromised or malnourished patients, and those draining large volumes of chyle, may benefit from early surgical intervention as the defect rarely closes spontaneously.

♦ Idiopathic chylothorax. Therapeutic thoracentesis and adoption of a low-fat diet with medium-chain triglycerides (MCT) may be adopted in an attempt to reduce chyle flow. This is often of limited success, as the diet is often unpalatable and does not reduce chyle flow as effectively as a fasting state and total parenteral nutrition (TPN). However, resolution occurs in up to 80% of compliant patients.

♦ Other strategies include:

  • Octreotide, a somatostatin analogue, has been reported in paediatric series to enhance thoracic duct closure and reduce chyle production. The exact mechanism of action remains unclear; it probably includes reduction of intestinal fat absorption (mainly triglycerides), an increase in faecal fat excretion, and a possible attenuating effect on thoracic duct lymph flow.

- Image-guided percutaneous thoracic duct embolization may be attempted before surgical thoracic duct ligation is considered. This offers a minimally invasive treatment for patients unfit for surgery.
- VATS or thoracotomy allows ligation, over-sewing or fibrin glue application to try and achieve surgical closure of a thoracic duct defect.

Case 28

A previously fit and well 23-year-old banker was admitted on the acute medical take with an 8-week history of progressive exertional breathlessness, worse over the preceding 3 days. He also reported a brief episode of central pleuritic chest pain on the day of admission.

On admission his oxygen saturation was 91% at rest on air. His pulse was 100bpm and BP 101/59. His JVP was visible (+3cm). His calves were soft and non-tender and his chest clear.

Investigations

- Full blood count, U&E and liver function were within normal limits
- INR 1.3, troponin I 0.8
- ABG on air, pH 7.4, $PaCO_2$ 3.0kPa, PaO_2 7.8kPa, $[HCO_3]^-$ 24.5mmol/L, BE −0.95mmol/L
- ECG, sinus tachycardia 110bpm with anterior T wave inversion
- His CXR and CT pulmonary angiogram are shown in Fig. 28.1.

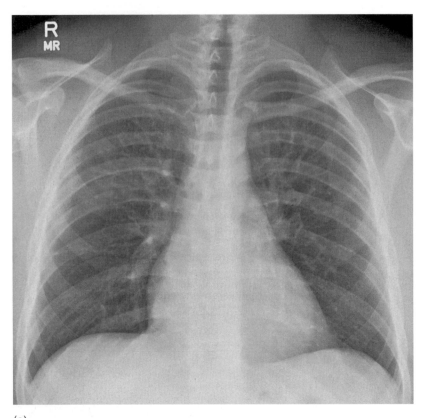

(a)

Fig. 28.1 (a) CXR

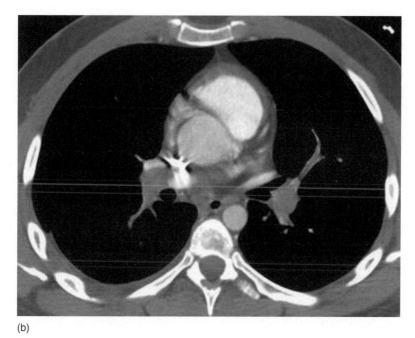

(b)

Fig. 28.1 (b) CT pulmonary angiogram.

Questions

28a) What does the CXR show (Fig. 28.1a)?

28b) What is the diagnosis?

Answers

28a) **What does the CXR show (Fig. 28.1a)?**

There is mild cardiomegaly with either upper lobe blood vessel pre-dominance, or lower zone oligaemia. His right costophrenic angle is blunted.

28b) **What is the diagnosis?**

Extensive bilateral pulmonary emboli are demonstrated on the CT pulmonary angiogram. The right lower and middle lobe pulmonary arteries were completely occluded. There was also evidence of right ventricular strain, i.e. RV (right ventricle, measured at the level of the tricuspid valve) to LV (left ventricle, measured at the level of the mitral valve) diameter ratio >1 (see Fig. 28.2). An RV to LV diameter ratio >1 is also suggestive of severe PE and associated with a more than three-fold increase in risk of intensive care admission (Araoz *et al.* 2003), and death. Evidence of RV strain on CTPA has a sensitivity of approximately 78–92% and specificity of 100% for the presence of RV dysfunction, when compared to echocardiographic findings (Ghaye *et al.* 2006).

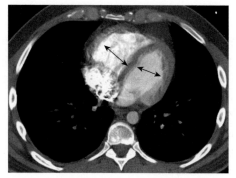

Fig. 28.2 CT pulmonary angiogram. RV 4.6cm: LV 4.2cm, ratio >1 (arrows denote site of measurement for calculation of the RV:LV ratio).

Progress

The patient was admitted to the ward and started on a therapeutic dose of low molecular weight heparin and warfarin treatment. However, on day two he became more breathless.

On examination he was anxious and oxygen-dependent with SaO$_2$ on 100% oxygen of 97% (86% on air). He had a persisting tachycardia, >115bpm, BP 120/70 and tachypnoea (>25 per minute).

Investigations

- ABG on 100% oxygen, pH 7.45, PaCO$_2$ 4.7kPa, PaO$_2$ 14.7kPa.
- Trans-thoracic echocardiography: normal left ventricular function, dyskinetic septum, and a dilated right ventricle with mild-moderately impaired function. The aortic valve was bicuspid, with root dilatation, and the estimated pulmonary artery pressure was 30mmHg (including the CVP in mmHg).
- Doppler ultrasound of both legs showed no evidence of proximal DVT.

Questions

28c) Should the results of these tests alter your management?

28d) How and when would you assess risk for future thrombo-embolic events?

28e) Is thrombolysis indicated?

Answers

28c) Should the results of these tests alter your management?

No. This patient has had a sub-massive PE with evidence of right ventricular dysfunction on echocardiography. Treatment with anticoagulation is appropriate—therapeutic dose low molecular weight heparin should be administered initially and oral anticoagulation (usually warfarin) commenced at the same time. Heparin should be continued for at least 5 days (the time needed to ensure reduction in the vitamin K-dependent clotting factors affected by warfarin) and then discontinued once the international normalized ratio (INR) has been >2 for 48h.

Echocardiographic findings aid prognostication for patients with PE but do not form part of the routine acute assessment. However, RV hypokinesia is present in 40% of those with a systolic blood pressure >90mmHg and impaired RV function is an independent predictor of mortality at 90 days. Persistent pulmonary hypertension (after 6 weeks), a patent foramen ovale (>4mm) and mobile right-heart thrombus are all recognized markers of a poor prognosis.

Raised troponin concentrations indicate myocardial injury and indicate a group at higher risk of death. In one study, elevation of troponin I >1.5ng was associated with RV dysfunction and increased mortality rates.

Other potential prognostic markers in PE include:

- Brain natriuretic peptide (BNP)—levels are higher in those with PE, particularly with RV impairment, and may be predictive of adverse outcome.
- Heart-type fatty acid binding protein (H-FABP) has been mooted as a promising early marker of RV damage in acute PE (Puls *et al.* 2007).

28d) How and when would you assess risk for future thrombo-embolic events?

There is currently no consensus concerning who to screen for thrombophilia disorders following venous thrombo-embolism (VTE). An individual approach should be taken, with routine screening for occult malignancy not recommended. However, testicular examination in a young male with VTE, prostate specific antigen (PSA) measurement in older men and a breast examination in female patient are prudent.

Screening would be appropriate for patients:

- Age <50y with spontaneous VTE
- With recurrent thrombosis
- With a family history of VTE
- With VTE in association with pregnancy or use of oral contraceptive
- Unusual site of VTE (e.g. sagittal sinus, axillary, mesenteric, portal)
- With history of warfarin induced skin necrosis.

Testing should be performed at least 2 weeks, and preferably one month, *after completing anticoagulation* because:

- Antithrombin concentrations, and occasionally protein C and S levels, can be reduced in acute thrombosis
- Antithrombin levels can be reduced by heparin use
- Warfarin reduces functional activity of protein C and S, and can falsely raise antithrombin levels

However, factor V Leiden, prothrombin gene mutations and the presence of antiphospholipid antibodies can be screened for at any time.

28e) **Is thrombolysis indicated?**

The use of thrombolysis in submassive PE is controversial. At present the only indication for use of thrombolytic therapy in PE is a clinically massive event with haemodynamic instability (systolic BP <90mmHg, or a fall of 40mmHg for 15 minutes not due to other causes). Some clinicians consider refractory hypotension or hypoxaemia, and right ventricular dysfunction appropriate indications for thrombolysis (Konstantinides *et al.* 2002); however, national guidelines do not support its use in these settings.

Progress

On day 3, despite continuous high-flow oxygen, the patient became increasingly agitated and distressed. CPAP was commenced on the High Dependency Unit and oxygen saturations maintained around 90% with 7cmH$_2$0 and inspired oxygen concentrations of 85%.

Investigations

- HR 134, BP 110/65
- ABG on CPAP 7cmH$_2$0, FiO$_2$ 0.85: pH 7.50, PaCO$_2$ 4.3kPa, PaO$_2$ 8.84kPa, SaO$_2$ 91%, [HCO$_3$]$^-$ 24.3mmol/L, BE −1.6mmol/L
- INR 2.0
- CXR no new changes.

Questions

28f) Discuss the pros and cons of the following treatment options:
- Discuss with cardiothoracic surgeons possible embolectomy
- Proceed to endotracheal intubation
- Perform medical thrombolysis
- Insert an inferior vena caval (IVC) filter.

Answer

28f) **Discuss the pros and cons of the following treatment options:**
- **Discuss with cardiothoracic surgeons possible embolectomy**
- **Proceed to endotracheal intubation**
- **Perform medical thrombolysis**
- **Insert an inferior vena caval (IVC) filter.**

- Surgical embolectomy, catheter embolectomy or clot fragmentation is neither widely available nor recommended in submassive PE. However, in massive PE, if thrombolysis is contraindicated or haemodynamic instability persists, the case should be discussed with the local cardiothoracic team. There are no randomized controlled trials comparing efficacy of surgical intervention versus thrombolytic therapy in submassive PE.

- Full resuscitation should be performed in all patients with full intensive care support, including invasive ventilation and inotropes, if required.

- There is no evidence to suggest improvement of clinical outcome with the addition of thrombolytic therapy to standard treatment in patients with submassive PE. However, in patients with massive PE i.e. with signs of haemodynamic instability, without absolute contraindication, thrombolysis should be administered.

- In non-massive PE, IVC filter placement reduces the rate of recurrence, but has no impact on overall mortality, and increases the incidence of subsequent deep vein thrombosis. Insertion should be considered for patients with massive PE when potential additional emboli might be catastrophic.

Progress

The cardiothoracic surgical team did not recommend surgical embolectomy and thrombolysis was performed with rt-PA. An immediate improvement with reduced oxygen demand (PaO_2 34kPa on 60% oxygen) and resolution of dyspnoea was seen. However, a few hours later he suddenly deteriorated and became unresponsive following a witnessed *grand mal* seizure. On examination he had evidence of a left hemisphere stroke.

Question

28g) What do you think has happened?

Answer

28g) **What do you think has happened?**

He could either have suffered a cerebral haemorrhage secondary to the thrombolysis, or had a cerebral infarction as a result of paradoxical emboli through a pre-existing intra-cardiac shunt, e.g. patent foramen ovale (PFO) or atrial septal defect (ASD).

Progress

He was intubated and ventilated. A CT brain showed left-middle cerebral artery infarction with oedema and resultant mid-line shift. A trans-oesophageal echocardiogram showed reduction in the PAP (40mmHg) but revealed a patent foramen ovale. Further neurological decline occurred and following discussion with the patient's family active treatments were stopped.

Conclusion

This case demonstrates a delayed paradoxical embolism through a patent PFO in a young man who received thrombolysis for a PE. A PFO is present in up to 26% of people on autopsy and is often associated with a poor prognosis and higher mortality in patients with PE. As a consequence of raised right-sided heart pressures, due to the PE, the PFO would have opened allowing right-to-left intra-cardiac shunting (increasing an already elevated A-a gradient) and paradoxical embolization of the thrombus resulting in the catastrophic outcome seen here.

The role of thrombolysis in non-massive PE remains controversial. Current guidelines do not recommend its use.

Further reading

Araoz PA, Gotway MB, Trowbridge RL, Bailey RA, Auerbach AD, Reddy GP (2003). Helical CT pulmonary angiography predictors of in-hospital morbidity and mortality in patients with acute pulmonary embolism. *J Thorac Imaging*; **18**: 207–216.

Dong BR, Yue J, Liu GJ, Wang Q, Wu T (2006). Thrombolytic therapy for pulmonary embolism. *Cochrane Database of Systematic Reviews*; **2**: CD004437.

Ghaye B, Ghuysen A, Bruyere PJ, D'Orio V, Dondelinger RF (2006). Can CT pulmonary angiography allow assessment of severity and prognosis in patients presenting with pulmonary embolism? What the radiologist needs to know. *Radiographics*; **26**: 23–39.

Konstantinides S (2002). The case for thrombolysis in acute major pulmonary embolism: hemodynamic benefits and beyond. *Intensive Care Med*; **28**: 1547–1551.

Puls M, Dellas C, Lankeit M, Olschewski M, Binder L, Geibel A (2007). Heart-type fatty acid-binding protein permits early risk stratification of pulmonary embolism. *Eur Heart J*; **28**: 224–229.

Tapson VF (2008). Acute pulmonary embolism. *N Engl.J Med*; **358**: 1037–1052.

Case 29

A 17-year-old adolescent was referred for optimization of exercise-induced asthma control. His complaints were of exercise-induced dyspnoea, cough, wheeze and choking episodes during competitive sport, particularly rugby. On three occasions his symptoms were so severe that an ambulance was called. The patient reported that the crew had said he was very wheezy and oxygen relieved his symptoms, but he was not admitted to hospital. Symptoms were unrelieved by inhaled salbutamol taken before and after exercise. He had no nocturnal symptoms, and other daytime activities were not restricted. He had been diagnosed with asthma by his GP 6 months previously, and at the time of review was taking combined salmeterol and fluticasone at a dose of 250µg fluticasone, two puffs twice daily. This had failed to control his symptoms. Examination was normal.

Investigations

- Hb 13.2×10^9/L, WCC 8.4×10^9/L (eosinophils 0.25×10^9/L), platelets 365×10^9/L
- Total IgE 47kU/L, precipitating serum IgG antibodies to *Aspergillus fumigatus* negative, *Aspergillus*-specific IgE < 0.35KU/L
- Peak flow in clinic 520L/m (90% predicted), serial peak flow chart kept for preceding 3 weeks showed no evidence of diurnal variability. CXR normal.
- Pulmonary function is shown in Table 29.1.

Table 29.1 Pulmonary function tests

	Measured	% Predicted
FEV_1(L)	4.1	108
FVC(L)	5.0	116
FEV_1/FVC	82	
RV(L)	1.6	138
TLC(L)	6.7	116
VA(L)	6.2	121
TL_{CO}(mmol/min/kPa)	12.64	117
K_{CO}(mmol/min/kPa/L)	2.04	97

Questions

29a) What features are in favour or against the diagnosis of exercise-induced asthma?

29b) What would be the most appropriate next investigation?

Answers

29a) **What features are in favour or against the diagnosis of exercise-induced asthma?**

The diagnosis of exercise-induced asthma cannot be made with certainty at present, primarily given the lack of improved symptoms with a short-acting bronchodilator. Exercise-induced asthma can be present in the absence of asthma symptoms at other times. The absence of objective measures of poor (conventional) asthma control (lack of PEFR variability, or demonstrable airflow obstruction) does not exclude exercise-induced asthma. The patient has been taking a moderate dose of inhaled corticosteroid (ICS) with a long-acting bronchodilator. ICS usually reduce the severity of exercise-induced asthma symptoms, but these can still occur, even when there is adequate control of daytime symptoms and normal resting measures of airway calibre. Salmeterol gives good protection against exercise-induced asthma, but its long onset of action requires it to be taken at least 30 minutes (optimally 2.5h) before exercise. Also, regular use of salmeterol as a preventative measure for exercise-induced asthma is associated with development of tolerance to its protective effect. From the data presented, the only objective support for exercise-induced asthma is the isolated finding of air-trapping (RV 138% predicted, versus TLC 116% predicted) suggesting possible mild chronic airflow limitation.

29b) **What would be the most appropriate next investigation?**

Exercise testing with lung function would be the most appropriate next investigation. The type of exercise testing will vary depending on local availability, but it is important that the intensity of exercise in the laboratory mirrors that in the field, and standardized conditions are recommended (e.g. FEV_1 measurement pre-exercise and 1, 3, 5, 7, 10, 15 and 20 minutes post-exercise). Other measures of airway inflammation, such as sputum eosinophil quantification or a methacholine challenge, are unlikely to be helpful in clarifying the nature of the exercise induced symptoms.

Progress

Exercise testing was performed, which recreated his symptoms. Post-exercise spirometry and flow-volume loop are shown in Table 29.2.

Table 29.2

Minutes post-exercise	FEV₁ (L)	PEFR (L/min)
0	3.9	510
1	3.8	510
2	3.75	490
3	3.7	500
5	3.8	490
8	3.7	500
20	3.8	480

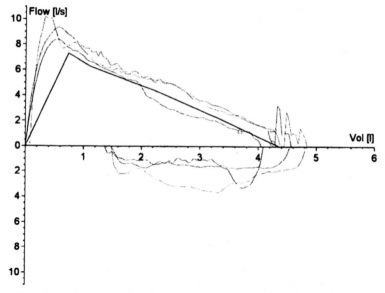

Fig. 29.1 Flow volume loop showing three breaths at peak exercise. Expiration upwards, inspiration downwards, TLC far left of graph. Darker line is approximate predicted normal expiratory curve.

Questions

29c) Interpret the exercise lung function data.

29d) What is the diagnosis?

29e) What management steps would you institute?

Answers

29c) **Interpret the exercise lung function data.**

The exercise spirometry shows no significant drop in either FEV_1 or PEFR to support the diagnosis of exercise-induced asthma. A fall of > 10% is considered abnormal and is used as a cut-off for diagnosis of exercise-induced asthma.

The flow volume loop demonstrates severe truncation of the inspiratory limb with normal appearances of the expiratory limb, suggesting extra-thoracic upper airways obstruction, most likely from the glottis.

29d) **What is the diagnosis?**

Exercise-induced vocal cord dysfunction. In vocal cord dysfunction (VCD) there is abnormal movement of the vocal cords during respiration (usually, but not uniformly, in inspiration) causing a number of symptoms, most commonly dyspnoea, stridor (which was the 'wheeze' described by our patient), choking, throat tightness and cough.

The pathophysiology is unclear but probably involves interaction between laryngeal hyper-responsiveness, possible inflammatory insults or emotional triggers, and autonomic imbalance leading to symptoms. VCD has been described in association with exercise and in elite athletes where diagnosis may require specific testing with the particular sporting activity, rather than in the lung function lab. The gold standard for diagnosis is visualization by laryngoscopy of abnormal adduction of the anterior two-thirds of the vocal cords with the creation of a posterior glottic 'chink'. This is usually needed during symptoms, as the cords are frequently normal between attacks. Asthma and psychiatric morbidity are frequent associations of VCD. In one of the largest series of VCD patients, asthma was present in over 50% and 73% had a major psychiatric disorder. On further questioning it was clear there was a significant psychological burden on this patient, with the death of his half- brother 6 months previously, stress from pending school exams and caring for his second disabled brother.

29e) **What management steps would you institute?**

There are no randomized, controlled trials of treatment for VCD. Most case series of VCD describe the beneficial effect of speech therapy, but other forms of breathing retraining, such as can be delivered by a respiratory physiotherapist, may be of value. Psychological assessment may be helpful. Withdrawal of medication for previously presumed diagnoses (especially asthma) is important if these are excluded. In the acute setting, success has been reported with Heliox (21% O_2, 79% helium); this response may help in diagnosis also, given that reduction in airflow resistance would only be expected at sites of turbulent flow such as across a narrow laryngeal chink.

Further reading

Anderson S, Brannan J (2001). Exercise induced asthma. In: O'Byrne PM and Thomson NC (eds). *Manual of Asthma Management* (2nd edn). Saunders, London, chapter 36, pp. 471–486.

Ayers J, Gabbott PL (2002). Vocal cord dysfunction and laryngeal hyperresponsiveness: a function of altered autonomic balance? *Thorax*; **57**: 284–285.

McFadden ER Jr, Zawadski DK (1996). Vocal cord dysfunction masquerading as exercise-induced asthma. a physiologic cause for 'choking' during athletic activities. *AJRCCM*; **153**: 942–947.

Newman KB, Mason UG, Schmaling KB (1995). Clinical features of vocal cord dysfunction. *AJRCCM*; **152**: 1382–1386.

Case 30

A 29-year-old lawyer, 16 weeks pregnant, presented with cough, wheeze and dyspnoea on exertion; she had also required antibiotics for repeated chest infections and lost 15kg in weight since her previous pregnancy 2 years previously. At that time she had been diagnosed with asthma when she also had shortness of breath. This had responded well to salbutamol and beclomethasone and, in retrospect, there had been previous episodes of self-limiting cough and wheeze over several years.

She had had a normal CXR a year previously. There were no pets at home and she was taking combined salmeterol and flixotide via a spacer. She had not had any oral steroids recently.

On examination she was pale and tachycardic. There were crackles and wheezes throughout the chest.

Investigations

- SaO_2, 98%
- FEV_1, 2.4L (80% predicted normal)
- VC, 2.9L (83% predicted normal)
- FEV_1/VC ratio, 83%
- Hb, 11.7g/dL
- MCV, 89.5fL
- Neutrophils, 6.21×10^9/L
- Lymphocytes, 1.03×10^9/L
- Eosinophils, 0.86×10^9/L
- CRP, 159mg/L
- ESR, 89mm/h
- Sputum, profuse growth of *Streptococcus pneumoniae*
- ANA/ANCA, negative
- CXR, declined, as pregnant
- Urinalysis, negative
- Free thyroxine, 14.6pmol/L (11.5–22.7)
- Renal function, normal.

Question

30a) What are the most likely diagnoses?

Answer

30a) **What are the most likely diagnoses?**

Asthma is the most likely diagnosis, given the previous history of salbutamol and beclomethasone responsive wheeze. Her normal spirometry is a little unexpected given the wheeze on examination, but she was using inhaled bronchodilators and steroids regularly. There is clear evidence of superadded infection with crackles, raised CRP and profuse *Streptococcus pneumoniae* in the sputum.

Progress

She was treated with 14 days of amoxicillin, continuing inhaled salmeterol and flixotide (oral steroids were not considered necessary), making a moderately rapid recovery. Two weeks later she had fully recovered.

Investigations

- Neutrophils, 4.73×10^9/L
- Lymphocytes, 1.86×10^9/L
- Eosinophils, 1.35×10^9/L
- CRP, 24mg/L, falling to <8 one month later
- ESR, 51mm/h
- ANA/ANCA, negative.

The rest of her pregnancy was uneventful apart from another chest infection with cough, fever, chest pain and wheeze; the sputum grew a fully sensitive *Haemophilus influenzae* and she responded to amoxicillin.

Progress

Two months post-partum she presented again with malaise, fever, night sweats, weight loss, haemoptysis, cough and wheeze. She had had a brief episode of whole body urticaria, a few itchy cutaneous nodules and a small sub-lingual ulcer with raised edges.

Investigations

- SaO_2, 90%
- Hb, 13.4g/dL
- Platelets, 669×10^9/L
- Neutrophils, 8.43×10^9/L

- Lymphocytes, 2.75×10^9/L
- Eosinophils, 5.33×10^9/L
- CRP, 182mg/L
- ESR, 96mm/h
- ANA/ANCA, negative
- *Aspergillus*, negative precipitins
- Urinalysis, normal
- Renal function, normal
- Total IgE, 451kU/l (5–120)
- Sputum, profuse growth of *Haemophilus influenzae* and *Moraxella catarrhalis*
- CXR Fig. 30.1.

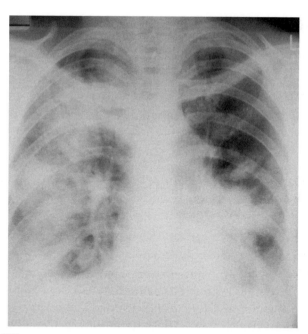

Fig. 30.1 CXR.

Questions

30b) What additional diagnosis should now be considered?

30c) Which features support, and which do not, this additional diagnosis?

Answers

30b) **What additional diagnosis should now be considered?**

Churg Strauss syndrome (CSS) or other eosinophilic lung disease.

30c) **Which features support, and which do not, this additional diagnosis?**

The eosinophil count is over 10 times the upper limit of normal, and is unlikely to be due to asthma alone. Levels in excess of 1.5 times normal are usually seen in CSS. The elevated inflammatory markers would be compatible with infection alone.

Cutaneous features are seen in up to 80% of patients with CSS, e.g. urticaria and subcutaneous nodules. Fever and weight loss are equally common. The tongue base ulcer could be vasculitic, but there is limited other evidence of active vasculitis. Urinalysis showed no blood or protein and the blood markers of vasculitides were negative, renal involvement can be absent in over 50% of cases of CSS. Other recognised complications of CSS, such as sinusitis, rhinitis, mono-neuritis multiplex, and pericarditis, were absent.

Progress

The patient declined a bronchoscopy. An HRCT scan was considered insufficiently likely to alter management to justify exposing her to the significant extra risks of irradiating lactating breast tissue. A dose of 40mg of oral prednisolone produced a dramatic clinical response within days, the SaO_2 rose to 98%, and the CXR, CRP and ESR returned to normal within a month. The eosinophil count fell to 0.23×10^9/L within a week, and 0.08×10^9/L within 2 months.

Over the subsequent year her steroid dose fluctuated, but rarely went below 10 mg/day. She had repeated sputum-positive chest infections that responded rapidly to antibiotics. Her steroid dose was slowly reduced to 5mg/day.

Six months later, her systemic symptoms returned with an eosinophil count of 7.7. Urinalysis was positive for blood and protein (although renal function remained normal). ANA and ANCA remained negative. FEV_1/VC was 3.5L/3.8L (>100% predicted). Prednisolone was increased to 50 mg a day.

Questions

30d) Should this further development surprise you?

30e) What further tests might be helpful?

30f) What alternative disease-modifying therapies might be considered?

30g) What additional medications should be considered?

30h) Compare the repeat spirometry with that done originally, what does this suggest might have been present the first time?

30i) What is the likely prognosis?

Answers

30d) **Should this further development surprise you?**

No, the evolution of Churg Strauss (defined as asthma, hypereosinophilia and small vessel vasculitis with granuloma) in this patient is typical. It tends to be a three-phase disease. The initial phase is usually atopic asthma alone (with or without sinusitis/rhinitis). The second phase, months or a few years later, is associated with a rising eosinophil count; this is often the first clue that the problem is more than just asthma. A rising eosinophil count is probably more useful than a single raised value that can occur in asthma anyway, although >1.5 times normal is an accepted cut-off. The third phase is the onset of vasculitis, which again can be months or years later.

30e) **What further tests might be helpful?**

The diagnosis is fairly secure without further tests. The absence of a positive ANCA (or anti-myeloperoxidase, MPO) does not greatly reduce diagnostic confidence, as it is positive in only 40–70% of patients. A renal biopsy may be appropriate in doubtful cases (particularly if there is an abnormal urinary sediment), or biopsies from alternative sites of involvement, such as skin or upper airway lesions (in retrospect a biopsy of the tongue ulcer would have been easy and safe). Renal biopsy is likely to be abnormal in the presence of haematuria, and carries only a small risk; a focal, segmental, necrotizing glomerulonephritis is usually seen. Chronic eosinophilic pneumonia is an alternative diagnosis (see case 18) although a vasculitis is not seen; an apparent chronic eosinophilic pneumonia can evolve into CSS.

However, further investigations to detect other potentially serious complications should be done. ECG and cardiac ultrasound may detect coronary vasculitis, with pericarditis and heart failure, which contributes to about half the deaths. In the absence of relevant symptoms (diarrhoea, bleeding, abdominal pain) routine gastro-intestinal investigations are not necessary. If the diagnosis is secure, the response to steroids is classically rapid and further tests may be pointless and delay treatment.

30f) **What alternative disease-modifying therapies might be considered?**

The aggressiveness of 'remission-induction' therapy will depend on the severity and extent of the vasculitis, and may require additional immunosuppression with cyclophosphamide, particularly if there is significant renal, cerebral, gastro-intestinal or cardiac involvement. This is not often seen in Churg Strauss syndrome, compared to Wegener's granulomatosis, for example. However, steroid-sparing agents should be considered once remission has been achieved.

Potential immunosuppressants for maintenance therapy could be either daily azathioprine (with careful monitoring of white cell counts and liver function) or weekly methotrexate (with careful monitoring of bone marrow, liver and renal function). Disease activity can be monitored by symptoms, eosinophil count, urine haematuria/proteinuria, CRP and ESR. Specific markers, such as ANCA/anti-MPO, can remain high

VASCULITIS ACTIVITY SCORE 2003

O Tick box only if abnormality represents active disease (use the Vasculitis Damage Index, VDI to score items of damage). If there are no abnormalities in a system, please tick the "None" box

☐ If all the abnormalities recorded represent smouldering/low grade/ grumbling disease, and there are no new/worse features, please remember to tick the box at the bottom right corner

	None	Active disease		None	Active disease
1. General	O		**6. Cardiovascular**	O	
Myalgia		O	Loss of pulses		O
Arthralgia or arthritis		O	Valvular heart disease		O
Fever ≥ 38.0 °C		O	Pericarditis		O
Weight Loss ≥ 2 kg		O	Ischaemic cardiac pain		O
			Cardiomyopathy		O
2. Cutaneous	O		Congestive cardiac failure		O
Infarct		O	**7. Abdominal**	O	
Purpura		O			
Ulcer		O	Peritonitis		O
Gangrene		O	Bloody diarrhoea		O
Other skin vasculitis		O	Ischaemic abdominal pain		O
3. Mucous membranes/eyes	O		**8. Renal**	O	
Mouth ulcers/granulomata		O	Hypertension		O
Genital ulcers		O	Proteinuria >1+		O
Adnexal inflammation		O	Haematuria ≥10 rbc/hpf		O
Significant proptosis		O	Creatinine 125-249 µmol/l		O
Red eye (Epi)scleritis		O	Creatinine 250-499 µmol/l		O
Red eye conjunctivitis/ blepharitis/keratitis		O	Creatinine ≥ 500 µmol/l		O
Blurred vision		O	Rise in creatinine > 30% or		
Sudden visual loss		O	Creatinine clearance fall > 25%		O
Uveitis		O.	**9. Nervous system**	O	
Retinal vasculitis/retinal vessel Thrombosis/retinal exudates/			Headache		O
Retinal haemorrhages		O	Meningitis		O
			Organic confusion		O
4. ENT	O		Seizures (not hypertensive)		O
Bloody nasal discharge/nasal			Stroke		O
Crusts/ulcers and/or granulomata		O	Cord lesion		O
Paranasal sinus involvement		O	Cranial nerve palsy		O
Subglottic stenosis		O	Sensory peripheral neuropathy		O
Conductive hearing loss		O	Motor mononeuritis multiplex		O
Sensorineural hearing loss		O	**10. OTHER**	O	
					O
5. Chest	O				O
Wheeze		O			O
Nodules or cavities		O			O
Pleural effusion/pleurisy		O			
Infiltrate		O	**PERSISTENT DISEASE ONLY:**		
Endobronchial involvement		O			
Massive haemoptysis/Alveolar haemorrhage		O	Tick here if all the above abnormalities are due to low grade grumbling disease and not due to new/ worse disease	☐	
Respiratory failure		O			

Fig. 30.2 Birmingham vasculitis activity score (BVAS).

despite successful remission, and levels may also lag behind during an exacerbation.

Generic symptom and sign scores to assess vasculitis have been developed and are a useful *aide-mémoire* (Fig. 30.2).

30g) **What additional medications should be considered?**

Other therapies to consider are for bone protection, calcium and vitamin D, and/or biphosphonates.

30h) **Compare the repeat spirometry with that done originally, what does this suggest might have been present the first time?**

The improved spirometry indicates the original values were 'restrictive'. A CXR then would probably have had an infiltrate (infective or eosinophilic).

30i) **What is the likely prognosis?**

Overall 5-year survival rate is over 70% for Churg Strauss, better than Wegener's or microscopic polyangiitis. Relapse rates are about 20%. Complications of therapy can be more problematic than the disease itself.

Further reading

Brown K (2006). Pulmonary vasculitis. *Proc Am Thorac Soc*; **3**: 48–57.

D'Cruz DP, David P, Barnes NC (1999). Difficult asthma or Churg-Strauss syndrome? *BMJ*; **318**: 475–476.

Case 31

A 24-year-old female classroom assistant, who had immigrated to the UK from Pakistan 10 years previously, presented with a persistent productive cough, with yellow sputum, of 2 months' duration. She was 33 weeks pregnant. Auramine staining of three sputum samples revealed moderate numbers of acid fast bacilli.

Questions

31a) What would you do next?

31b) What are particular points you need to consider relevant to her pregnancy and subsequent delivery?

Answer

31a) **What would you do next?**

Management of open (infectious) pulmonary TB in this case requires close attention to several factors:

- Source case isolation. Segregation can be done out of hospital, if multi-drug resistant TB (MDR-TB) is not suspected, and cases are advised to remain in the confines of their home until 2 weeks of appropriate treatment have passed.

  Current NICE guidelines advise against unnecessary hospitalization. However, if admission is indicated (e.g. poor social arrangements), all patients with open pulmonary TB should be nursed separately from immunocompromised patients, either by admission to a single room on a separate ward, or in a negative pressure room on the same ward. Smear-positive TB patients usually rapidly become non-infectious on initiation of adequate treatment, despite presence of bacilli in the sputum as these may simply be dead organisms.

- Notification. All forms of *Mycobacterium tuberculosis* are compulsorily notifiable under the Public Health (Control of Disease) Act 1984, whereas non-tuberculous mycobacterial infections are not. The doctor who confirms the diagnosis, or makes the decision to treat, is legally responsible for notifying the Consultant in Communicable Disease Control (CCDC)—Health Protection Agency—in England and Wales, or the equivalent Director of Public Health in Scotland and Northern Ireland. It is also advisable to inform the local TB nurse specialist who will be responsible for contact tracing, monitoring of patient compliance, administering directly observed therapy (DOT), if necessary, and ensuring continuity of treatment. Notification also allows identification of epidemiological trends and outbreaks.

- Contact tracing. A complete and thorough contact investigation is important to protect contacts from progression to clinically active disease. The TB nurse specialist should initiate a cascade of testing to identify any persons exposed to the source case.

  Increasing duration and proximity of contact with an infectious case are key determinants of the likelihood of infection.

  Close contacts (e.g. family), and casual contacts exposed through the patient's work as a school classroom assistant, should be screened in accordance with the NICE guidelines. All contacts should initially have a Mantoux test if <35y and a CXR if >35y of age. Further investigations are prompted by whether the contact has had a BCG, together with the result of the Mantoux test (see NICE Clinical Guideline 33, March 2006).

• Clinical treatment. Quadruple therapy should be commenced whilst bacteriological sensitivities are awaited. (This patient has no risk factors for MDR-TB, i.e. previous treatment for TB, contact with known MDR-TB, HIV infection, failure of clinical response to treatment or prolonged sputum smear positivity).

A 6-month regimen comprising rifampicin (R), isoniazid (H), pyrazinamide (Z) and ethambutol (E) for 2 months followed by rifampicin and isoniazid for 4 months is advocated for respiratory disease.

The fundamental principle of initiating one bacteriocidal, and one bacteriostatic drug to which the mycobacteria are sensitive, still holds true. However, although initiation of three agents was previously accepted, the appreciation that current rates of resistance (approximately 10% to one drug) are increasing, has led to quadruple therapy being used routinely. Triple therapy (rifampicin, isoniazid and pyrazinamide) is seldom used, but may be implemented for patients (with no risk factors for MDR-TB) who are incapable of reporting visual changes which may arise as a consequence of the ethambutol (e.g. learning difficulties, young children). Triple therapy may also be considered if the mycobacteria are proven to be fully sensitive.

Combination tablets, dosage based on patients' weight, commonly Rifinah® (rifampicin/isoniazid) and Rifater® (rifampicin, isoniazid and pyrazinamide), may improve patient compliance.

31b) **What are particular points you need to consider relevant to her pregnancy and subsequent delivery?**

TB in pregnancy.

• None of the first-line medications have been shown to be teratogenic and treatment should be instituted with these agents.

• Second-line agents, such as streptomycin and other aminoglycosides, are best avoided if possible because of potential foetal ototoxicity.

• Breast-feeding is safe whilst on antituberculosis medications.

• Measurement of liver function tests should be performed prior to treatment in pregnancy, and post-partum. (Patients with pre-existing liver disease, risk factors for chronic liver disease, e.g. heavy alcohol intake, and HIV infection should also have pre-treatment tests of liver function performed.) There is no need to repeat tests during the treatment course unless clinically indicated (see question 31f).

◆ Babies of sputum-positive mothers should receive isoniazid prophylaxis for 6 weeks, if delivered within 2 weeks of the mother starting antituberculous medication. If a tuberculin skin test at this point is negative, the isoniazid can be stopped and the BCG given 1 week later.

◆ The efficacy of the BCG vaccine is debatable and in the UK is estimated to be 70–80% effective at reducing the chance of a child developing active disease. Few data suggest a benefit over the age of 16y. Neonates born in places where TB is widespread (notification rate >40 per 100,000), or with 1 or more parents or grandparents born in a high-incidence country, or with a family history of TB within 5 years, should be offered vaccination.

Progress

Quadruple anti-TB chemotherapy was commenced.

Three children from the class in which the patient worked had positive Mantoux reactions (8mm, 11mm and 15mm) following initial screening. Interferon-gamma tests were performed (ELISpot)—one child's result was negative, two were positive.

Questions

31c) What should the patient have been warned about, prior to initiation of the anti-TB medication?

31d) What is the significance of the negative interferon gamma assay? Does this child require chemoprophylaxis?

Answer

31c) **What should the patient have been warned about, prior to initiation of the anti-TB medication?**

The importance of compliance with medication should be stressed. The potential adverse effects of antituberculosis medication should be explained (they occur in approximately 10% of patients), although most are mild and do not necessitate discontinuation of treatment. They include:

◆ Red-orange discoloration of secretions (urine, stool, sweat, tears—contact lenses (may be permanently stained). Monitoring urinary discolouration can provide an indirect measure of patient compliance.

◆ Nausea, vomiting, diarrhoea, fever and anorexia.

◆ Patients should be advised to contact a doctor if they develop:
  • A rash (usually maculopapular but erythema multiforme can develop with isoniazid, and a photosensitivity reaction with pyrazinamide)
  • 'Flu-like' symptoms (rifampicin-induced)
  • Bruising (rarely blood dyscrasias arise as a result of isoniazid, and thrombocytopenia due to ethambutol).

◆ Patient should stop their medication and contact their doctor or TB specialist nurse urgently if they notice:
  • Jaundice
  • Visual disturbance—red/green colour blindness, blurring, loss of vision or pain (optic neuritis may be secondary to ethambutol 0.3%)
  • Peripheral sensory changes e.g. numbness (neuropathy rarely due to isoniazid).

◆ Rifampicin and isoniazid (and related compound preparations) are best absorbed on an empty stomach (half an hour before food). Pyrazinamide and ethambutol can be taken at any time.

◆ Drug interactions are common. Isoniazid is a liver enzyme inhibitor and increases the blood level of drugs metabolized by the liver. Rifampicin induces liver enzymes and thereby decreases the effectiveness of drugs metabolized hepatically, e.g. warfarin, contraceptive pill.

◆ Pyridoxine is given if there is a high risk of peripheral neuropathy, i.e. in diabetes, HIV infection, alcohol dependency or renal failure.

31d) **What is the significance of the negative interferon gamma assay? Does this child require chemoprophylaxis?**

The negative ELISpot result, indicates that the Mantoux response was a false-positive in this instance (probably representing prior vaccination, or exposure to environmental mycobacteria). If the child had had exposure to MTB, then an appropriate T cell response against the ESAT-6 and CFP-10 proteins from the organism would have been mounted, and a positive ELISpot seen. Further investigation is unnecessary in this child.

In the past, difficulties in determining the significance of a positive Mantoux tuberculin skin test (TST) were commonly encountered, i.e. whether it reflected active or latent *Mycobacterium tuberculosis* infection, or a response to either previous BCG administration, or environmental mycobacteria. (Since the tuberculin solution contains a crude mixture of >200 *Mycobacterium tuberculosis* proteins, of which some antigens are shared with other mycobacteria besides *Mycobacterium tuberculosis*.)

Recent advances in mycobacterial genomics have isolated two proteins— early secretory antigenic target-6 (ESAT-6) and culture filtrate protein-10 (CFP-10)—within a stretch of DNA (denoted *region of difference-1*) of *Mycobacterium tuberculosis*, which are *not* present in the BCG vaccination or environmental mycobacteria. These proteins are strong targets for T helper cells of patients with *Mycobacterium tuberculosis* infection. Measurement of the specific T-cell response to these antigens is now possible via an ELISpot assay (T-SPOT.TB; Oxford Immunotec) or enzyme-linked immunosorbent assay (ELISA—QuantiFERON-TB test; Cellestis). T cells from individuals with latent *Mycobacterium tuberculosis* infection become sensitized to ESAT-6 or CFP-10 *in vivo*; when the T cells re-encounter these antigens *ex vivo* in the overnight ELISpot or ELISA tests, they release a cytokine, interferon (IFN)-γ. In the ELISpot test, each sensitized T cell gives rise to a dark spot, which is counted by an automated reader. The ELISA test measures the IFN-γ concentration in the supernatant of a sample of diluted whole blood after 24h of incubation with ESAT-6 and CFP-10. The response is independent of the subject's BCG status. To date, the main use of these tests has been in the diagnosis of latent *Mycobacterium tuberculosis* infection, although further indications are being investigated.

Progress

In the two positive cases, both had normal clinical examinations and CXRs. Chemoprophylaxis was given with 3 months of rifampicin and isoniazid (an alternative is 6 months of isoniazid).

Four days later, the index patient re-presented with 24h of general malaise, nausea and anorexia. She had been compliant with her medication.

Question

31e) What would you do next?

Answer

31e) **What would you do next?**

Gastro-intestinal side effects of anti-TB medication are well recognized.

Initial advice to take the drugs with or after food may help to ease symptoms, as can administration at a different time of day, e.g. before going to bed rather than in the morning.

Liver function should be tested as non-specific gastro-intestinal symptoms may reflect drug induced hepatitis. (A pregnancy test should also be performed, if this is a possibility, in women of child-bearing age with persisting nausea.)

Progress

Repeat blood tests (day 4 of treatment) showed: Hb 9.4g/dL, MCV 71.7fL, WBC 7.8 × 10⁹/L, INR 1.1, bilirubin 10μmol/L, ALT 82IU/L, ALP 209IU/L, Alb 39g/L and CRP 82mg/L.

Despite taking the tablets with food over the next few days, her nausea worsened and she began to vomit. Concern regarding her poor oral intake was expressed by the obstetricians and she was admitted to hospital for intravenous fluids. Repeat blood tests (day 7) were performed.

Hb 10.4g/dl, WBC 9.2 × 10⁹/L, platelets 225 × 10⁹/L, INR 1.1, Urea 7.6mmol/L, Cr 58μmol/L, bilirubin 13μmol/L, ALT 431 IU/L, ALP 299 IU/L, Alb 37g/L.

Questions

31f) What is the most likely explanation for the abnormal LFTs?

31g) What would you do next?

- Stop the rifampicin
- Stop rifampicin and isoniazid
- Stop all the medication
- Stop the current medication and start an alternative anti-TB agent
- Continue the medication but repeat the blood tests in 1 week.

31h) How should she be managed in hospital?

Answers

31f) **What is the most likely explanation for the abnormal LFTs?**

A rise in hepatic transaminases is not uncommon following initiation of TB chemotherapy. Particular risk groups for derangement of liver function include those with known underlying liver disease, such as alcohol dependency, cirrhosis and hepatitis B or C, malnourished patients, and possibly the elderly, children and those taking herbal therapies.

Current recommendations suggest:

- If the AST or ALT rise is <2 × normal, repeat liver function at two weeks. If levels have fallen, further tests are only required if symptoms occur.
- If the repeat test shows levels ≥2 × normal, liver function should be monitored weekly for 2 weeks, then 2-weekly until normal.

If transaminase levels are ≥5 × normal, or ≥3 × normal with clinical symptoms (i.e. 'flu-like' symptoms, nausea, vomiting or anorexia), the rifampicin, isoniazid and pyrazinamide should be stopped. However, sustained treatment with a single agent should never occur.

Hepatitis serology, if clinically indicated, for co-existent viral hepatitis should be considered.

31g) **What would you do next?**

- **Stop the rifampicin**
- **Stop rifampicin and isoniazid**
- **Stop all the medication**
- **Stop the current medication and start an alternative anti-TB agent**
- **Continue the medication but repeat the blood tests in 1 week.**

In the case of smear-positive disease within 2 weeks of starting treatment, an alternative treatment should be given until liver function returns to normal. Close liaison with the local microbiology or infection control, or public health team, is prudent.

Streptomycin is often used for this indication alongside ethambutol. Newer agents to consider include fluoroquinolones (e.g. levofloxacin or moxifloxacin). In this case, at 33 weeks of pregnancy, the risks must be weighed against the need for treatment. The risk of potential foetal oto-toxicity is greatest from streptomycin (but is increased with all aminogly-cosides) and within the first trimester. If a patient becomes pregnant or is found to be pregnant whilst taking streptomycin, it should be discontinued, if possible. In this case, the risks of untreated disease outweighed those of streptomycin and this was commenced with ethambutol. Renal function monitoring is required.

31h) **How should she be managed in hospital?**

As this patient has received <2 weeks of treatment she is potentially infectious.

- Segregation from other patients is required until 2 weeks of treatment is complete. A face mask should be worn if she leaves isolation, i.e. to go to radiology or other areas where contact could be made with susceptible individuals (including young infants).

- Ideally all patients should be nursed in a negative pressure room. However, if on a ward with no immunosuppressed patients, a single room vented to the air outside would be suitable. If the ward had immunosuppressed patients or the risk of MDR-TB was high, a negative pressure room is essential.

- Staff and visitors should wear masks if in contact with patients with potential open pulmonary MDR-TB or where aerosol generating procedures, e.g. bronchoscopy or sputum induction techniques are being performed.

- Re-introduction of the medications. (This can be done without the need for alternative therapy, in the period awaiting return to normality of the liver function, if patients are smear negative or >2 weeks into their treatment course.) Incremental drug re-introduction strategies vary between different centres with no universally agreed approach. Several regimes add drugs every 3 days if the problem is fever, rash or vomiting; however, liver function derangement often takes longer to respond and requires longer intervals between escalation. Once liver function is normal, sequential introduction of the original drugs can be made with daily clinical review and liver function testing in the following order:

  - 1st: isoniazid 50mg/day, titrating up to 300 mg/day after 2–3 days if no reaction occurs, this is then continued. Isoniazid is postulated to induce hepatic injury via an idiosyncratic hypersensitivity reaction which may be dose-dependent. The exact mechanism, however, remains unclear, although it can safely be re-introduced once the liver function returns to baseline.

  - 2nd: after 2–3 days, if stable, rifampicin 75 mg/day can be started, increasing to 300 mg after 2–3 days if no deterioration. Reintroduction is safe, if liver function and clinical parameters remain normal. Serious liver injury is rare; however; rifampicin does increase the hepatotoxicity of isoniazid, probably via enzyme induction and elevation of toxic metabolite concentrations, which explains in part the reason for re-initiation of the latter agent first.

• Finally: pyrazinamide 250mg/ day, increasing to 1g after 2–3 days, and then to 1.5g (<50 kg) or 2g (>50kg). If the transaminases rise when pyrazinamide is restarted, the drug should be avoided as cases of potentially fatal hepatic necrosis have been reported.

• If there is no deterioration, the medication can be continued and the streptomycin stopped.

• If a further reaction occurs to pyrazinamide, then rifampicin and isoniazid for 9 months, with ethambutol for the initial 2 months, should be given.

Progress

Re-introduction of quadruple therapy was successful and, after 23 days in hospital, the patient was discharged. Her baby was born a week later and, following completion of 6 weeks of isoniazid syrup chemoprophylaxis, had a negative Mantoux test and received the BCG vaccination 7 days later.

Further reading

Control and prevention of tuberculosis in the United Kingdom: Code of Practice (2000). Joint Tuberculosis Committee of the British Thoracic Society. *Thorax*; **55**: 887–901.

Chemotherapy and management of tuberculosis in the United Kingdom: recommendations (1998). Joint Tuberculosis Committee of the British Thoracic Society. *Thorax*; **53**: 536–548.

Lalvani A (2007). Diagnosing tuberculosis infection in the 21st century: New tools to tackle an old enemy. *Chest*; **131**: 1898–1906.

Tuberculosis: Clinical Guideline 33 (March 2006). *National Institute for Health and Clinical Excellence (NICE)*. http://www.nice.org.uk/nicemedia/pdf/CG033FullGuideline.pdf (accessed 1st September 2009)

Case 32

A 66-year-old lady originally presented to the emergency department with gradual onset of shortness of breath over a week. The relevant past medical history was of asthma, and her father died post-operatively of a pulmonary embolus aged 59. She was very ill with signs of pulmonary hypertension with a loud P2, raised JVP, tachycardia and hypotension. Her right ankle was minimally swollen. ECG showed right bundle branch block and right axis deviation. Breathing air, the PaO_2 was 8.0kPa and the $PaCO_2$ was 3.4kPa, indicating a large alveolar to arterial gradient for oxygen (7.8kPa). Her pulmonary arteries were enlarged on CXR.

A clinical diagnosis of acute on chronic pulmonary emboli was made, and confirmed on ventilation/perfusion (V/Q) scanning with multiple and extensive unmatched perfusion defects. She was anti-coagulated and within a week her symptoms had greatly improved.

On review in clinic 1 month later, her exercise tolerance was partly back to normal and she was more troubled by cough. She had stopped her inhalers whilst in hospital and they had not been restarted. Anti-coagulation had been exemplary. On examination, all signs of pulmonary hypertension had resolved.

Investigations

- Lung function showed a mild obstructive picture and the SaO_2 was 92%.
- Repeat V/Q scan had improved, but showed persisting unmatched perfusion defects.
- A CT pulmonary angiogram 1 month later revealed a thrombus lying in the right main pulmonary artery but the rest of the pulmonary vasculature appeared normal, apart from a few sub-segmental emboli in the upper lobes.
- ECG showed resolution of the right-sided abnormalities.
- Cardiac echo showed a right ventricle at 3.9cm (upper limit of normal 3.0cm) with all other chambers normal. Estimation of the peak pulmonary artery pressure (PAP) was technically unsatisfactory, but reported as 90mmHg (upper limit of normal = 35mmHg).
- In view of the clinical improvement no further action was taken apart from recommending that the INR was kept between 2.5 and 3.0.

Progress

Six months later she returned to out-patients with some deterioration in her shortness of breath. She had lost 25kg in weight. She had experienced two episodes of central chest pain following exercise, in association with marked breathlessness and felt she was going to pass out. Warfarin control had been excellent.

On examination there was no evidence of pulmonary hypertension and her SaO_2 was now 96%. On walking 50m her heart rate rose to 105 and her SaO_2 fell to 86%, with mild shortness of breath. Repeat cardiac echo showed a moderately dilated right ventricle (3.3cm), moderately reduced systolic contraction and, again, the peak PAP was difficult to measure, but estimated to be about 100mmHg.

Investigations

Further tests were performed 10 months after the initial presentation to elucidate the cause of her continuing shortness of breath.

- Shuttle walking distance 150m, SaO_2 fell to 88%
- V/Q scan again showed multiple matched defects

Right-sided cardiac catheter data:

- Mean PAP, 29mmHg
- Normal right atrial pressure
- Cardiac output, 4.1L/m
- Mixed venous SO_2, 51%
- Following prostacyclin infusion, cardiac output rose to 5.5L/m.

Questions

32a) What is the most likely diagnosis, should any alternatives be considered?

32b) What might have been the cause of the chest pain and dizziness?

32c) Describe the catheterization data; does the discrepancy with the echo surprise you?

32d) What is the likely untreated prognosis for this patient?

32e) What forms of treatment are available at this stage?

Answers

32a) **What is the most likely diagnosis, should any alternatives be considered?**

The most likely diagnosis is chronic pulmonary thrombo-embolic pulmonary hypertension (CTEPH). The persisting unmatched Q scan perfusion defects strongly suggest this. The cardiac catheterization abnormalities are not very severe, and, therefore, other possible causes should be considered, including a return of her asthma, for example.

32b) **What might have been the cause of the chest pain and dizziness?**

If pulmonary hypertension is the cause of her chest pain and dizzyness, then right heart angina and a fall in cardiac output could be occurring on exercise, but is more often seen in primary pulmonary hypertension. Alternatively, if anxiety and hyperventilation were the cause, then they could be causing these symptoms, but the fall in SaO_2 on exercise clearly rules out hyperventilation syndrome (case 12).

32c) **Describe the catheterization data; does the discrepancy with the echo surprise you?**

The catheterization data show a mildly raised mean PAP (upper limit of normal about 25mmHg). The cardiac output is slightly reduced, but the mixed venous SO_2 is curiously low and does not seem compatible with the SaO_2 and the cardiac output. The echo measurement of PAP is the peak pressure (systolic) and, therefore, higher than the mean pressure. The echo method relies on the conversion of the peak velocity of a regurgitant tricuspid valve jet during systole into a theoretical peak PAP—this is not always accurate and significant discrepancies occur.

32d) **What is the likely untreated prognosis for this patient?**

Untreated, the prognosis is not clear. Most pulmonary emboli resolve quickly on treatment with anti-coagulation. Disappearance of extensive clots within a week has been reported but recent series have shown that over half have detectable residual defects at 3 months. Non-resolution is associated with gradual deterioration of exercise tolerance and a rise in PAP, after an apparent 'honeymoon' period. The conventionally quoted incidence of this is about 0.5% after an episode of acute pulmonary emboli. However, in one recent study, the prevalence of an abnormally high PAP (>40mmHg systolic and >25mmHg mean) was 1% at 6 months, 3% at 1 year and 4% at 2 years, with no further increase thereafter. Once this process of a persistent and rising pressure is established, it is believed that progression to death is almost inevitable without treatment. Prognosis correlates with current PAP; a 50% 10-year survival with mean pressures between 30 and 40mmHg, but only a 20% 2-year survival if the pressure is over 50mmHg.

32e) **What forms of treatment are available at this stage?**

Treatment consists mainly of maintaining adequate anti-coagulation and the use of pulmonary-specific vasodilators. Choice of vasodilators used to be based on the results of acute studies but these do not accurately predict long-term response and, in practice, various drugs are tried. Calcium channel blockers are used extensively. Long-term oxygen may have a role, even in mild hypoxia.

The mechanism of progression from acute emboli to a chronic deteriorating condition is not understood. There are probably three components. First, there may be *in situ* extension of clot with gradual silting up of the pulmonary tree, although resected specimens show organized thrombi, all of similar age, suggesting little new thrombus is forming. Second, the raised PAP may cause remodelling of the distal vascular bed with an increase in vascular resistance, as is thought to occur in other causes of pulmonary hypertension. Third, if there is significant hypoxia, then this may also provoke further, and eventually irreversible, rises in vascular resistance. Abnormalities of fibrinolysis or thrombotic tendency have not been consistently found in these individuals. The factors about the patient that tip the process from resolution to progression are unclear, although a previous embolus, younger age, more severe initial embolic event, poor resolution of the Q scan perfusion defects and a higher PAP acutely, all seem to predict higher risk. Some cases have not had a recognizable acute embolic event.

Further investigations and progress

Conventional pulmonary angiography showed multiple obstructed lobar and segmental arteries in the right lung, but the left side was largely clear of emboli.

A Greenfield IVC filter was introduced and she was placed on amlodipine 5mg/day. The evidence for a benefit from such IVC filters in this situation is very limited.

By 18 months post-presentation, her shuttle walking distance had fallen to 360m, SaO_2 falling to 89%, but she denied any deterioration in her day-to-day activity levels. Repeat cardiac catheterization showed a mean PAP of 63mmHg.

At 25 months her PAP was 43mmHg, cardiac output 5.4L/m. No pulmonary vasodilation occurred following nitric oxide (NO) inhalation.

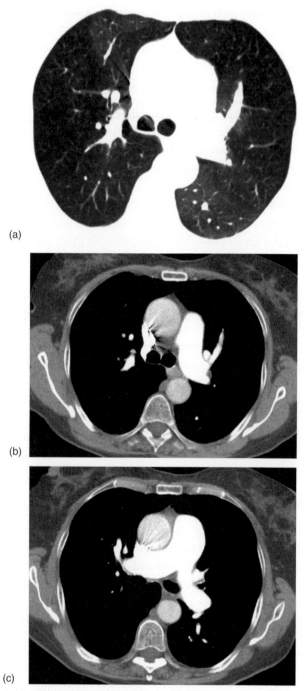

Fig. 32.1 (a)–(c) CT pulmonary angiograms.

Echocardiography 3 years post-presentation showed a right ventricular diameter of 4.2cm and an estimated peak PAP of about 100mmHg.

Shortly after this she complained of increased SOB and occasional morning haemoptysis. She was now visibly cyanosed at rest (SaO$_2$ 92%), had a raised JVP (+5cm) with a dominant V wave, loud pulmonary second sound, parasternal heave and a right ventricular 3rd sound; ECG showed right ventricular hypertrophy. Echo again gave a peak PAP estimate over 100mmHg. Shuttle walking distance was 430m with the SaO$_2$ dropping to 84%. Overnight oxygen levels were stable at about 83–85%, overnight oxygen via nasal prongs was prescribed.

Questions

32f) What further treatment options are there for this lady?

32g) What further imaging is required before considering this treatment?

32h) Does the CTPA (Fig. 32.1) suggest this treatment would be appropriate?

32i) What is the main risk of this treatment?

32j) What would you do?

32k) Could anything have been done to prevent this complication occurring at the time of the original pulmonary embolus?

Answers

32f) **What further treatment options are there for this lady?**

Further attempts to lower PAP could include the newer pulmonary artery vasodilators, including prostacyclin analogues (epoprostenol, beraprost, iloprost), endothelin receptor antagonists (bosentan, sitaxsentan, ambrisentan) and phospho-diesterase-5 inhibitors (sildenafil), although not all these drugs are licensed for this purpose. Preliminary evidence (no RCTs) suggests they lower PAP and improve exercise tolerance. The most successful therapy, in a carefully selected subgroup, is pulmonary thrombo-endarterectomy. Organized thrombi in main and lobar vessels are removed by careful dissection along a plain between the arterial wall and the occluding mass. Skilled surgeons can extend the endarterectomy into segmental level. Surgical success clearly depends on skill and experience.

32g) **What further imaging is required before considering this treatment?**

Surgical success also depends on there being significant resectable organized thrombus, rather than more distal secondary vascular changes, as the cause for the increased vascular resistance. Pulmonary angiography, preferably conventional as well as MRI, helps define the resectable tissue. In addition, Q scans may help; with significant thrombi the scan shows

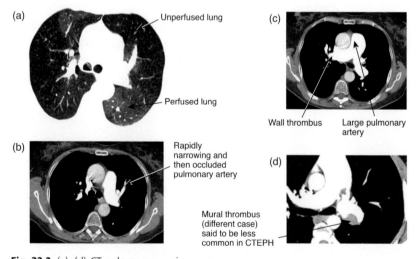

Fig. 32.2 (a)–(d) CT pulmonary angiograms.

clear segmental defects; with secondary distal vascular changes, the Q scan abnormalities tend to be very much more diffuse. However, there is a considerable degree of subjectivity in the interpretation of these scans.

32h) **Does the CTPA (Fig. 32.1) suggest this treatment would be appropriate?**

The CTPA (Fig. 32.1) shows several things. The first slice (a, lung windows) shows mosaic perfusion of the lung, implying defects of perfusion, compatible with blocked pulmonary arteries. The second slice (b) shows sudden narrowing of a left pulmonary arterial branch and then sudden cessation, probably due to occlusion. The third slice (c) is very hard to interpret but shows a large main pulmonary trunk (bigger than the aorta) and probable organized thrombus lining the right proximal pulmonary arteries, which in theory could be resectable. The angiographic appearance of resectable disease results from the complex interplay between occlusion and recanalization. Thus chronic thrombi appear different to acute thrombi, with webs traversing lumina, intimal irregularities, pouch-like defects, abrupt narrowing of vessels, often at branch origins, and the absence of apparent intraluminal filling defects.

32i) **What is the main risk of this treatment?**

Thrombo-endarterectomy carries a significant in hospital mortality, approximately 5–20%, depending on centre and surgeon experience. Risk is increased in those over 70, obesity, co-morbid disease (e.g. COPD, ischaemic heart disease and renal failure), right ventricular failure (i.e. raised right atrial pressures) and possibly the duration of pulmonary hypertension. The main immediate complication is re-perfusion pulmonary oedema, perhaps similar to high altitude pulmonary oedema. Following removal of the thrombus, PAP may remain higher than normal and feed through to unprotected capillaries leading to wall damage, pulmonary oedema and haemorrhage.

32j) **What would you do?**

The operative decision is difficult given the unpredictable rate of decline, uncertainty over operability and the immediate in-hospital mortality.

32k) **Could anything have been done to prevent this complication occurring at the time of the original pulmonary embolus?**

The place of thrombolysis in acute massive PE, in the absence of circulatory compromise, is not yet established. There is little evidence that thrombolysis of big clots will reduce progression to CTEPH.

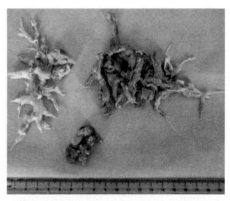

Fig. 32.3 Thrombo-endarterectomy specimens, from a different case, removed during surgery (courtesy of Dr Keith McNeil).

Further progress

Five years post-presentation this lady had a pulmonary artery thrombo-endarterectomy (Fig. 32.3) after a repeat conventional pulmonary angiogram had suggested the prospect of a good result.

Three months post-operatively her resting saturations were normal at 98% on air. Shuttle walk was 420m with a drop in SaO_2 to 92%. Echo showed unchanged right ventricular dimensions, and there was no tricuspid regurgitation to estimate pressures.

Six months post-operatively (5½ years after her initial PEs), mean PAP was measured directly at 18mmHg.

Ten years post-presentation, and 5 years post-operatively, shuttle walking distance was 560m, resting SaO_2 96%, and remained at 96% on exercise. Echo-derived peak PAP was 34mmHg (at the upper limit of normal).

This is a remarkable result and increasingly this is the outcome of thrombo-endarterectomy in carefully selected cases of CTEPH performed in highly specialized centres.

Further reading

McNeil K, Dunning J (2007). Chronic thrombo-embolic pulmonary hypertension (CTEPH). *Heart*; **93**: 1152–1158.

Pengo V, Lensing AW, Prins MH, Marchiori A, Davidson BL, Tiozzo F *et al.* (2004). Thrombo-embolic Pulmonary Hypertension Study Group Incidence of chronic thromboembolic pulmonary hypertension after pulmonary embolism. *N Engl J Med*; 350: 2257–2264.

Segovia Cubero J, Ortiz Uribe JC, Gómez Bueno M, Moñivas Palomero V, González González M, Alonso-Pulpón Rivera L (2007). Role of bosentan in patients with chronic venous thrombo-embolic pulmonary hypertension. *Med Clin (Barc)*; **128**: 12–144.

Case 33

A 71-year-old lady was referred to the respiratory clinic with a history of non-resolving pneumonia. She had presented to her GP 3 weeks previously with cough, fevers and myalgia, and despite courses of amoxicillin and erythromycin, she was not improving. On direct questioning, there was a 3-month history of progressive dyspnoea and a dry cough. She had been seen by her GP four times over the last 6 months and treated with antibiotics for chest infections on each occasion.

Her past history included controlled epilepsy, and bilateral knee replacements for osteoarthritis several years ago. She was a lifelong non-smoker with pigeons living in her roof space, but with no other personal or family history of note. Her current medication included phenytoin, paracetamol and diclofenac.

On examination she was sweaty, although afebrile. She was tachypnoeic (22/min) at rest, her oxygen saturations were 93% and on examination of the chest she had bilateral fine crackles at the bases with no other signs of cardiac decompensation.

Routine blood tests

+ Hb, 13.9g/dL
+ WCC, 15.4×10^9/L
+ Platelets, 315×10^9/L
+ Neutrophilia, no eosinophilia
+ Urea and electrolytes normal
+ CRP, 57mg/L
+ ESR, 43mm/h.

Pulmonary function tests

FEV$_1$/(L)	1.42 L	(75% predicted)
FVC (L)	1.87L	(79% predicted)
FEV$_1$/FVC ratio	76%	

CXRs from 2 months ago (a) and from this episode (b) are shown in Fig. 33.1.

(a) 2 months previously

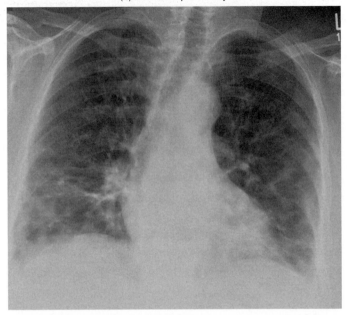

(b) Current

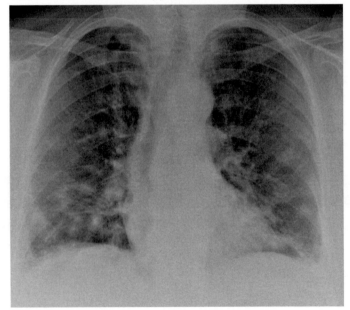

Fig. 33.1 CXRs

Questions

33a) Interpret the CXRs (Fig. 33.1a and b).

33b) What is the differential diagnosis?

33c) Justify your choice for the next two most relevant investigations.

aaaaaaaok...

Answers

33a) Interpret the CXRs (Fig. 33.1a and b).

The CXRs show bilateral multifocal consolidation. This appears to be worse in the current CXR (Fig. 33.1b) compared to 2 months ago (Fig. 33.1a). The infiltrates appear to show a lower zone and peripheral predominance. In addition, these changes are observed in the context of radiologically preserved lung volumes (i.e. no volume loss).

33b) What is the differential diagnosis?

The differential diagnosis is that of multifocal consolidation. In this specific case, infection with pneumonoccous or 'typical' bacterial pneumonia is an unlikely cause—the timeframe is too long and the CXR is not consistent (with bilateral changes and non-resolution despite appropriate antibiotic therapy). Certain forms of infective pneumonia should be considered in this context (e.g. *Mycoplasma*, *Coxiella*, *Psittacosis*). TB and atypical mycobacteria are a possibility and she is in a high-risk group; the elderly and immunosuppressed can present atypically. However, given her presentation with malaise in association with pulmonary infiltrates, cryptogenic organizing pneumonia (COP), eosinophilic pneumonia and vasculitis should be considered. In addition, given her history of seizures, chronic aspiration may be a possible cause as may drug-induced lung disease.

33c) Justify your choice for the next two most relevant investigations.

An HRCT chest is the investigation of choice, and will provide important information on differential diagnosis. It would be important to assess her peripheral eosinophil count, as this may change the likely diagnosis to include one of the lung infiltrate eosinophilic syndromes (see case 18) (although not all of these disease entities are associated with a peripheral blood eosinophilia). Further tests for autoimmune disease may be required, but it would be sensible to establish the pulmonary diagnosis first. A bronchoscopy with BAL would be a reasonable investigation, should there be doubt about the radiological pattern on CT, permitting exclusion of infective and malignant disease. Bronchoalveolar carcinoma (BAC) is a possibility, however the clinical presentation is inconsistent with this diagnosis

Progress

The patient proceeded to HRCT (see Fig. 33.2).

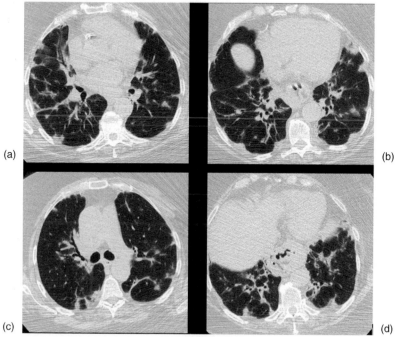

Fig. 33.2 (a)–(d) HRCT chest.

Questions

33d) Describe the HRCT findings (Fig. 33.2).

33e) What is the most likely diagnosis and why?

33f) Describe the histology that is associated with this condition.

33g) How would you investigate this patient further?

Answers

33d) Describe the HRCT findings (Fig. 33.2).

There are areas of ground glass and consolidation in all CT slices shown (Fig. 33.2), which appear to be predominant (in the lower slices, b and d) in a subpleural distribution. On the lowest slice (Fig. 33.3), the consolidation is centred around the associated bronchus (i.e. 'bronchocentric'). There are a few small nodules and the bronchial walls appear thickened and dilated. There is a marked absence of other changes, specifically there does not appear to be any areas of fibrosis (e.g. no traction dilatation of the airways) or gross lymphadenopathy.

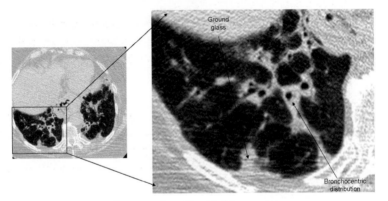

Fig. 33.3 Enlarged area of CT scan from Fig. 33.2d.

33e) What is the most likely diagnosis and why?

The most likely diagnosis is cryptogenic organizing pneumonia (COP), due to the combination of clinical and radiological features. Typical features of COP are as follows:

- Presentation. COP typically presents as a flu-like or infective illness, and is often misdiagnosed and treated as bacterial pneumonia with repeated courses of antibiotic therapy. Typical symptoms at presentation include respiratory symptoms (cough and shortness of breath) but also constitutional symptoms (malaise, fatigue, sweats, fevers and weight loss (seen in over 50% of cases). COP is not smoking-related.

- Radiology. Bilateral diffuse alveolar opacification in the presence of normal lung volumes (as seen here) is typical. Evidence of chronic fibrosis ('honeycombing') is usually not observed at presentation. However, several different radiological patterns are recognized including:

- 'Typical COP'—multiple alveolar shadows
- 'Focal COP'—a solitary opacity
- 'Infiltrative COP'—infiltrative appearing opacities
- Migratory infiltrates over time
- Peripheral infiltrate predominant
- Cavitation and pleural effusion are rarely seen.

The CT appearances are usually characteristic, although differentiation from eosinophilic lung disease, drug induced lung disease and carcinoma may not be possible.

- ◆ Other tests. As seen here, an associated increase in inflammatory markers is the norm, but is non-specific. Auto-antibodies are typically negative. Lung function typically shows mild to moderate restriction, and impairment of gas exchange manifested as a resting hypoxia and a widened Aa gradient.

- ◆ Differential diagnosis. Organizing pneumonia may be primary (cryptogenic) or secondary and can be associated with malignancy or connective tissue disease (especially polymyositis/dermatomyositis). Although COP is the most likely diagnosis, other possibilities in this case include:

  - Bacterial infection—this is unlikely in this case, as the history is of several months, the changes are bilateral and progressive and there has been no response to reasonable therapy.

  - Eosinophilic pneumonia—(see case 18) bilateral symmetrical infiltrates raises the possibility, but a more peripheral distribution and associated peripheral eosinophilia would be expected.

  - Hypersensitivity pneumonitis (HP)—(see case 8) the radiological appearance on CXR and CT is not typical here (acutely, HP would produce diffuse ground glass and centrilobar nodules, whereas chronically fibrosis would be seen). There is a potential antigen (the pigeons in the loft), so this should be considered and excluded.

  - Drug-induced lung disease—this patient is on anti-epileptics, which are a recognized cause of lung disease. However, there are no new or recently introduced medications and, although drug-induced disease may take on a variety of radiological patterns including the one seen here, this seems unlikely.

- Interstitial lung disease associated with connective tissue disease—there are, again, no pointers toward a co-existing connective tissue disease; however, the possibility should be considered and investigated. Most commonly, a UIP-type picture of lung disease is seen in association with connective tissue disease; however, COP is reported in association.
- Acute lung injury—in the absence of a clear precipitant, this is unlikely here.

33f) **Describe the histology that is associated with this condition.**

COP produces a distinct histopathological pattern, which is characterized by proliferation of granulation tissue within the small airways ('intraluminal buds'), associated with chronic alveolar inflammation (hence a bronchocentric pattern is seen on CT). This combination is referred to as 'organizing pneumonia'. Fibrosis and lung destruction is typically absent, as is vasculitis or granuloma formation.

On histology, organizing pneumonia with obliterative bronchiolitis may be seen in the context of several interstitial diseases—the absence of histological evidence of other disease within the same biopsy specimen suggests the diagnosis of COP.

33g) **How would you investigate this patient further?**

Investigations are guided by the above differential diagnosis. Establishing a diagnosis relies on a combination of clinical and radiological features, and may require histopathological confirmation. To narrow the differential diagnosis:

- A thorough history (including possible HP antigens, new medication and symptoms of a CTD) should be taken
- Blood eosinophil count should be measured
- Auto-antibodies may be reasonable, if there is a question of an associated CTD (e.g. anti-Jo1 especially in the context of myalgia)
- Bronchoalveolar lavage is a useful investigation to exclude other causes, specifically infection or malignancy (in the presence of an atypical radiological pattern, e.g. BAC); BAL findings are not specific to COP (e.g. increased cellularity, foamy macrophages, etc.) and therefore are not useful solely for diagnosis
- Transbronchial biopsies—please see below.

Progress

The patient proceeded to transbronchial biopsy (TBB), which showed clear evidence of organizing pneumonia and obliterative bronchiolitis, and no evidence of infection or granuloma formation.

Questions

33h) Discuss the pros and cons of further attempts at tissue diagnosis.

33i)   Describe treatment options and prognosis.

Answers

33h) **Discuss the pros and cons of further attempts at tissue diagnosis.**

Lung histology—there is some debate as to whether lung histology (i.e. at open or VATS lung biopsy) is always required for diagnosis. Obtaining lung histology (on larger sections of lung than is provided by TBB) is aimed at confidently excluding other pathological processes (e.g. NSIP, eosinophilic pneumonia, vasculitis). This is relevant to COP, as the pathological lesion (described in 33f) may be present in a number of non-COP lung diseases, and TBBs alone may not exclude these entities.

However, the risks of lung biopsy should be considered, as many of these patients are hypoxic at presentation, although this is not usually severe. Given that COP is generally very treatment responsive (see below), in the presence of supportive TBB results, a course of treatment may be used as a therapeutic and diagnostic strategy. Some authorities in the UK would therefore treat a typical case having excluded other diagnoses (e.g. by TBB) on the basis of typical clinical and radiographic appearances rather than insisting on lung biopsy.

A diagnosis of COP often commits patients to months of steroid therapy, with all the associated risks and potential complications. Depending on the case in question, it may be reasonable to treat initially without histological confirmation and proceed to biopsy in the case of unresponsive or relapsed disease.

33i) **Describe treatment options and prognosis.**

COP rarely recedes untreated and generally responds well to corticosteroids, although there are no robust studies assessing treatment in this area. A reasonable regimen is as follows:

- 0.5 to 1.5mg/kg prednisolone once per day for 4 to 8 weeks
- Gradual decrease in dose, if stable over the next 4 to 6 weeks, as tolerated to 0.5 mg/kg
- If remains stable, gradual reduction of dose to 0 over 3 to 6 months.

Optimal duration of therapy is not known, but is usually required for at least 3 and up to 12 months. During this period, the patient should be reviewed regularly to assess for radiological or clinical relapse requiring an increase in steroid therapy. Other immunosuppressants have been advocated in those unresponsive or intolerant of steroid therapy, but no evidence exists to inform clinical decision-making.

Rapid and full recovery occurs in the majority of patients on steroid therapy within a few weeks. If relapse off treatment does occur, this does not appear to be associated with long-term reduction in lung function or functional deficit. Overall, around one-third of patients will experience persistent disease that may require prolonged treatment. Relapse will commonly occur on withdrawal of steroid therapy, and these patients should continue to be monitored as out-patients, once symptoms and radiology have improved for several months.

In rapidly progressive, aggressive disease (fulminant COP), high-dose intravenous steroid has been recommended.

Further reading

ATS/ERS Statement (2002): International Multidisciplinary Consensus Classification of Idiopathic Interstitial Pneumonias: http://www.thoracic.org/sections/publications/statements/pages/respiratory-disease-adults/idio02.html (accessed 3rd September 2009)

BTS guidelines on interstitial lung disease (2008): http://www.brit-thoracic.org.uk/clinicalinformation/interstitiallungdiseasesDPLD/interstitiallungdiseaseDPLDguideline/tabid/126/default.aspx (accessed 3rd September 2009)

Cordier JF (2006). Cryptogenic organising Pneumonia. *Eur Respir J*; **28**: 422–446.

Case 34

A 36-year-old man with cystic fibrosis (CF) had small volume haemoptysis of 5–10ml every 3–4 days for 4 months. He was able to cycle short distances daily, although desaturated from SaO_2 92% at rest to 70% on walking. His other medical history was of gall stones, pancreatic insufficiency (on Creon) and CF related diabetes (on insulin). He had 3–4 infective exacerbations per year requiring intra-venous antibiotics.

He underwent a rapid deterioration and was admitted acutely via the emergency department with massive haemoptysis, coughing up 600ml blood over the course of 2h. He became haemodynamically unstable, with a heart rate of 150bpm and BP 70/45, and was drowsy. He had had increased sputum purulence for the preceding few days.

Investigations

Blood tests:

- Hb, 12.1g/dL
- CRP, 157mg/L
- MCV, 82fL
- Urea, 6.8mmol/L
- Platelets, 534×10^9/L
- Creatinine, 76μm/L
- WCC, 21.5×10^9/L (neutrophilia)
- Electrolytes, normal
- Clotting screen, normal.

Spirometry at previous out-patient visit:

- FEV_1 1.0L (22% predicted: steady decline from 1.75L 8 years ago)
- FVC 2.5L.

Recent sputum cultures:

- Moderate *Staphylococcus aureus*, sensitive to flucloxacillin
- Moderate *Pseudomonas aeruginosa* sensitive to ceftazadime, gentamycin and colistin.

See also Table 34.1 and Fig. 34.1.

Table 34.1 Arterial blood gases

	During current illness:	Previous sample when well:
FiO_2	0.40	0.21
pH	7.02	7.39
PaO_2	16.6kPa	7.9kPa
$PaCO_2$	20.8kPa	8.0kPa
SaO_2	96%	92%
Base excess	2.4mM/L	8.6mM/L
Bicarbonate	27mM/L	33mM/L
Lactate	1.5mM/L	

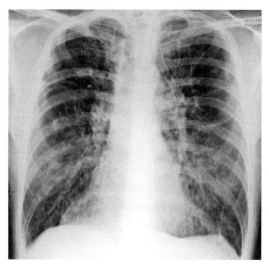

Fig. 34.1 CXR.

Questions

34a) Interpret the investigations outlined above.

34b) What risk factors for massive haemoptysis does this man have?

34c) What is the commonest mechanism of haemoptysis in patients with cystic fibrosis?

34d) Describe crucial steps in his immediate management in the emergency department (specialist procedures will be discussed later).

Answers

34a) **Interpret the investigations outlined above.**

Interpretation of investigations:

+ Arterial blood gases show a profound respiratory acidosis, and partial loss of his previously observed compensating metabolic alkalosis. The loss of metabolic compensation with a bicarbonate near normal, when previously high, is likely to be due to hypoxia, hypovolaemia and hypotension, causing lactate and other metabolic acid production.

+ Blood tests show haemoglobin is only marginally reduced and MCV is normal, in keeping with the acute history of this bleed. Inflammatory markers are all raised (CRP, white cell count and platelets) in keeping with active infection or an acute phase response.

+ Spirometry reflects severe obstructive airways disease, with a progressive decline over time.

+ Recent sputum cultures are positive for *Staphyloccus aureus* and *Pseudomonas aeruginosa*. These commonly represent long-standing colonization in CF; however, the increased sputum purulence may be due to current infection. Acute-phase reactants are non-specific, as they may be elevated in the presence of a large bleed. Recent microbiological cultures are often helpful in guiding preliminary treatment before current cultures are available.

+ The CXR shows extensive bronchiectatic changes throughout both lungs. There is a large cystic area in the left apex (Fig. 34.2), which on

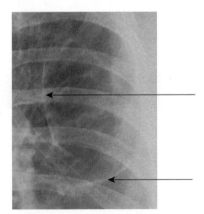

Fig. 34.2 Portion of CXR, with arrows indicating the medial and inferior walls of the large cystic area in the left apex.

comparison with previous films was not new. This particular CXR is not helpful in identifying the site of bleeding.

34b) What risk factors for massive haemoptysis does this man have?

Small-volume haemoptysis is extremely common in CF. The incidence of massive haemoptysis, as in this case, is less common at around 1 in 100 patients per year, and is defined as an acute bleed >240ml per 24h, or recurrent bleeding greater than 100ml/day over several days. Specific risk factors that this man has are:

- Older age, relative to the CF population. Median age for massive haemoptysis is 23 years, with only ¼ patients being <18 years old.
- More advanced disease: 61% of patients have an FEV_1 <40% predicted, although it can occur in patients with normal lung function.
- Declining lung function.
- *Staphyloccoccus aureus* and possibly *Pseudomonas* infection.

34c) What is the commonest mechanism of haemoptysis in patients with cystic fibrosis?

The commonest mechanism of massive haemoptysis is rupture of a bronchial artery with passage of blood into an airway. The underlying pathogenesis is thought to be due to persistent airway infection and inflammation. The chronic inflammation leads to proliferation of the bronchial vasculature through bronchial artery hypertrophy and angiogenesis. It has been hypothesized that virulence factors of *S. aureus* can lead to alterations in the pulmonary epithelium and vascular endothelium to stimulate bronchial artery proliferation. This results in a system of enlarged, dilated and tortuous vessels with collaterals and bronchopulmonary anastomoses.

Haemoptysis originates from the bronchial circulation in 90% of cases, and has the propensity to cause massive haemoptysis as bronchial arteries usually arise directly from the aorta, and therefore carry blood at systemic pressure. The bronchial circulation supplies conducting airways down to the terminal bronchioles, and most of this blood is carried away from the lung via the pulmonary veins. The flow through the bronchial circulation is a mere fraction of that through the pulmonary circulation, and the lung can function fairly well without it, example.g. following lung transplantation.

Bleeding from the pulmonary circulation or alveoli is much less common.

34d) **Describe crucial steps in his immediate management in the emergency department (specialist procedures will be discussed later).**

This man is critically unwell. His airway is at risk due to haemoptysis and drowsiness, putting him as risk of aspiration. He is hypoventilating with hypercapnic respiratory failure, and he has cardiovascular instability with hypotension due to blood loss. He requires urgent resuscitation, including:

- Intubation to protect his airway, to enable mechanical ventilation and to enable bronchoscopy, if required.

- Suctioning of secretions and blood may be helpful, although vigorous chest physiotherapy should be avoided until haemoptysis has settled. He will require admission to an intensive care unit.

- Volume replacement with vigilant fluid balance assessment is required.

- Intra-venous antibiotics as pulmonary infection contributes to on-going haemoptysis. In his case they should initially cover *Staphyloccus* and *Pseudomonas*, even though it is not entirely clear whether these represent infection or colonization. Repeat sputum cultures should be sent to enable the antibiotic spectrum to be narrowed in due course. Note that, although sputum cultures are not helpful in most respiratory disease, they form an essential part of management of patients with cystic fibrosis or bronchiectasis, enabling appropriate antibiotic choice.

- Position with bleeding side down to prevent aspiration into the unaffected lung, if the side of the bleed is known.

- Nebulized epinephrine (3–5ml 1:1000) may be of benefit, although is unproven for large bleeds.

- Tranexamic acid can be considered; it is an anti-fibrinolytic agent and synthetic derivative of the amino acid lysine that during clot formation binds reversibly to plasminogen, blocking its binding to fibrin and subsequent activation to plasmin. This results in the stabilization of clots by inhibition of tissue fibrinolysis. It may be given orally for recurrent small volume haemoptysis, although its role is massive haemoptysis is uncertain.

- Intra-venous vasopressin or subcutaneous/intra-venous octreotide have also been used, although caution is advised in patients with coexistent coronary artery disease or hypertension.

Questions

34e) What vitamin deficiency should be sought in massive haemoptysis in cystic fibrosis?

34f) What further investigation and interventional procedures should be considered?

Answers

34e) **What vitamin deficiency should be sought in massive haemoptysis in cystic fibrosis?**

Patients with cystic fibrosis may have a vitamin-K deficiency related to fat malabsorption and antibiotic usage, so studies should include coagulation profiles.

34f) **What further investigation and interventional procedures should be considered?**

A pulmonary angiogram and bronchial arterial embolization is recommended after an episode of massive haemoptysis, even if it settles. The bleeding bronchial artery is identified through extravasation of dye if bleeding is ongoing, visualization of tortuous vessels of increased calibre or aneurysmal dilatation. In this man's case, angiography showed hypervascularity and an aberrant systemic arterial supply to the lungs. A large anomalous bronchial artery arising from the left thyrocervical trunk descended through the mediastinum to feed a markedly hypertrophied left bronchial artery. This bronchial artery was embolized with polyvinyl alcohol. Alternative agents are foam granules (500–700μm in diameter) or platinum coils. Sometimes it is hard to identify the culprit vessel, and many advocate that all large and suspicious bronchial arteries should be embolized. Bronchial artery embolization has been found to be safe and effective in controlling the immediate bleeding (96% within 24h); however, the recurrence rates are greater than 50% within 4 months. Technical failure may arise due to non-bronchial artery collaterals from other systemic vessels.

Bronchoscopy should be considered for localization of the bleeding site, and to allow therapeutic intervention. Installation of 1:20,000 epinephrine may help control bleeding, although its role in massive haemoptysis is uncertain. Isolation of a bleeding segment with a balloon catheter allows lobar or segmental tamponade and may prevent aspiration of blood into the large airways. A 4-7 French 200cm balloon catheter is passed through the working channel of the bronchoscope, and may be left *in situ* for up to 24h. Leaving it in too long may lead to post-obstructive pneumonia or ischaemic mucosal injury. This is just a temporary measure until more definitive measures, such as embolization, can be used.

If bleeding can be localized to the right or left lung, unilateral lung intubation and selective ventilation may help protect the non-bleeding lung. For right-sided bleeding, a bronchoscope may be directed into the left main bronchus, which can then be selectively intubated using the bronchoscope as a 'guide wire' with the patient lying in the right-lateral position. The left lung is then protected from aspiration and selectively ventilated. For a left-sided bleeding source, the patient is placed in the left-lateral position and selective intubation of the right lung may be performed, but this may lead to occlusion of the right-upper lobe bronchus. Alternatively, the endotracheal tube may be passed into the trachea, and a Fogarty catheter (size 14 French/100cm length) may then be passed through the vocal cords beside the endotracheal tube, directed by the bronchoscope into the left main bronchus and inflated. This prevents aspiration of blood from the left lung and the endotracheal tube positioned into the trachea allows ventilation of the unaffected right lung. An alternative strategy for unilateral bleeding is to pass a double lumen endotracheal tube, which allows isolation and ventilation of the normal lung and prevents aspiration from the side involved by bleeding. This should only be performed by experienced operators to avoid the serious consequences of poor positioning.

Surgical resection may be carried out as a last resort for intractable bleeding from a localized site; however, the patient must be fit enough to withstand both the acute procedure, and the loss of lung function afterwards. It has a high mortality rate, approaching 50% in severely ill patients.

Outlook

A small, retrospective study compared patients who had had massive haemoptysis treated with embolization, with CF patients matched for age and FEV_1 who had not had haemoptysis or embolization. Over a period of up to 14 years, those with haemoptysis and embolization had a greater incidence of death (8/30 compared to 3/27) and lung transplant (9/30 compared with 1/27). They also had a numerically greater, though non-significant, increased incidence of infection with multi-drug resistant *Pseudomonas* and greater decline in FEV_1. 8/30 had recurrent major haemoptysis. The relative influence of infection, haemoptysis and the embolization process itself on lung function and outcome is not known.

The gentleman in this case made a remarkably good recovery from this particular episode. Unfortunately he went on to have recurrent massive haemoptysis and repeated embolizations, with step-wise deteriorations in lung function. He was referred and accepted for a lung transplant, but died of a further massive haemoptysis before this was possible.

Further reading

Graff GR (2000). Treatment of recurrent severe hemopytsis in cystic fibrosis with tranexamic acid. *Respiration*; **68**: 91–94.

Lordan JL, Gascoigne A, Corris PA (2003). The pulmonary physician in critical care. Illustrative case 7: assessment and management of massive haemoptysis. *Thorax*; **58**: 814–819.

Stenbit A, Flume PA (2008). Pulmonary complications in adult patients with cystic fibrosis. *Am J Med Sci*; **335** (1): 55–59.

Vidal V, Therasse E, Berthiaume Y, Bommart S, Giroux MF, Oliva VL *et al.* (2006). Bronchial artery embolization in adults with cystic fibrosis: impact on the clinical course and survival. *J Vasc Interv Radiol*; **17**: 953–958.

Case 35

A 37-year-old lady was referred to the chest clinic with a 6-week history of progressive shortness of breath, productive cough and malaise. She reported a several year history of productive cough, recurrent chest infections and repeated courses of antibiotics. She was known to have common variable immunodeficiency (CVID), which was diagnosed at the age of 19. She had undergone a splenectomy (for haemolytic anaemia) and received daily treatment with prophylactic penicillin and regular courses of intravenous immunoglobulin.

On examination, she was clubbed, tachypnoeic at rest (25/min) with oxygen saturations of 95% on room air. Chest examination revealed bibasal coarse crackles and a cough productive of whitish sputum. The CXR is shown in Fig. 35.1 and the pulmonary function in Table 35.1.

Lung function see Table 35.1

Table 35.1 Pulmonary function tests

	Measured	% Predicted
$FEV_1(L)$	2.3	80
FVC(L)	2.6	78
FEV_1/FVC %	87	
RV(L)	1.5	99
TLC(L)	4.2	85
TL_{CO}(mM/min/kPa)	6.14	71
K_{CO}(mM/min/kPa/L)	1.70	94

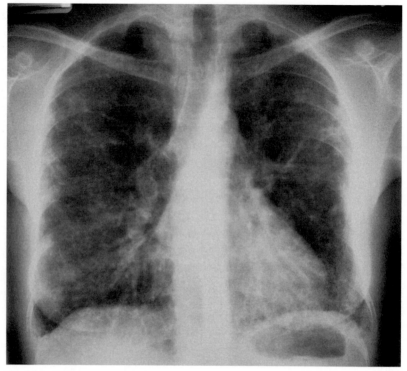

Fig. 35.1 CXR.

Questions

35a) Interpret the CXR (Fig. 35.1).

35b) Interpret the lung function (Table 35.1).

35c) What is the differential diagnosis in this case?

35d) What further investigations would be helpful?

Answers

35a) **Interpret the CXR (Fig. 35.1).**

The CXR shows bilateral mid- and lower-zone bronchial wall thickening with areas of reticulation peripherally. In addition, there are areas of nodular consolidation in the apices.

35b) **Interpret the lung function (Table 35.1).**

There is a restrictive defect (high FEV_1/FVC ratio, low FVC, low TLC) that is associated with a decreased gas transfer co-efficient. This is mainly due to the decrease in lung volume as K_{CO} is only minimally reduced.

35c) **What is the differential diagnosis in this case?**

The history of chronic sputum production, clubbing and radiological bronchial dilatation are suggestive of bronchiectasis (perhaps with inter-current infection given the infiltrates). However, lung function suggests a restrictive process (rather than obstruction, which would be more typical of bronchiectasis), and some of the CXR changes (nodular consolidation, peripheral fibrosis) are atypical for bronchiectasis alone and are suggestive of an additional process.

CVID is a disease associated with hypogammaglobulinaemia, recurrent bacterial infections and a number of immunological abnormalities. In the context of CVID, several associated lung pathologies are reported:

- Recurrent rhinosinusitis
- Recurrent lower respiratory tract infections
- Bronchiectasis
- Lymphoid tissue proliferation in the lung
- Malignancy (particularly primary lung lymphoma)
- Lymphocytic interstitial pneumonia.

35d) **What further investigations would be helpful?**

A high-resolution CT is probably the most useful next investigation, to assess for bronchiectasis and the presence of interstitial lung disease and consolidation. Sputum cultures are likely to be required given the presentation and underlying disease (possibility of atypical bacterial infection, including mycobacteria). Bronchoscopy and broncho-alveolar lavage are useful to exclude intercurrent infection, and may identify a predominant cell type (e.g. lymphocytes), which may suggest a specific diagnosis.

Progress

Blood tests revealed mildly raised inflammatory markers (CRP = 47mg/L, ESR = 41mm/h) and a raised white cell count (12.4×10^9/L, 70% neutrophils). Sputum cultures showed a profuse growth of *Pseudomonas aeruginosa* (PsA).

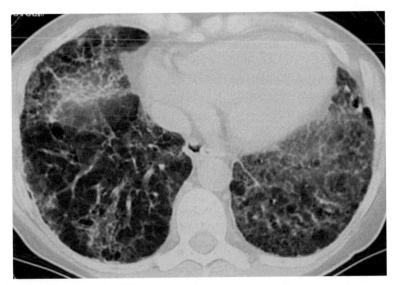

Fig. 35.2 High-resolution CT.

Questions

35e) Describe the CT findings.

35f) What diagnosis or diagnoses do they support?

35g) How would you investigate and manage this patient?

Answers

35e) **Describe the CT findings.**

The CT (Fig. 35.2 and 35.3) demonstrates some bronchiectasis in association with chronic fibrotic disease, and multiple areas of peripheral consolidation. In addition there are areas of ground glass attenuation (see Fig. 35.3).

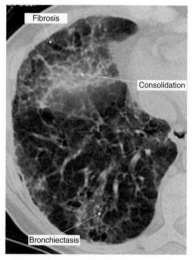

Fig. 35.3 Expanded portion of HRCT from Fig. 35.2.

35f) **What diagnosis or diagnoses do they support?**

The diagnoses supported by this HRCT scan are of bronchiectasis in addition to a cause of multi-focal consolidation. The differential diagnosis in this context must include typical and atypical infections (including mycobacterial and fungal disease), lymphoid interstitial pneumonia, pulmonary lymphoma and drug reactions.

35g) **How would you investigate and manage this patient?**

Bronchiectasis. The bronchiectasis is likely to have been caused by recurrent infections in the past due to CVID (inadequate host defence in the bronchial tree). The patient's clinical condition has deteriorated in the context of a positive sputum culture (PsA) and in this context, this should probably be treated with a view to microbiological eradication (4–6 weeks of oral ciprofloxacin with inhaled antibiotic). Some authorities would argue for an even more aggressive treatment strategy, as this is the first isolate of PsA and the patient was unwell (i.e. single or dual intravenous treatment to achieve eradication).

Chronic infection with *Pseudomonas* is seen in up to one-third of patients with bronchiectasis, and has been associated with poorer lung function, decreased quality of life and more frequent hospital admissions. The correct treatment paradigm in non-CF bronchiectasis is debated, with randomized evidence demonstrating good bacterial clearance using a combination of oral ciprofloxacin plus inhaled tobramycin for 14 days. However, this improvement in microbiology was not found to be associated with clinical improvement, and in fact a worsening of lung function was observed in these patients (presumably a reflection of airway response to inhaled therapy). Extrapolating data from the CF population, most clinicians would attempt eradication of *Pseudomonas* in non-CF bronchiectasis after the first isolate, although direct evidence is lacking. BTS guidelines on this subject are due to be published in 2009.

Further well-established treatments for bronchiectasis include chest physiotherapy, patient education, microbiology directed antibiotics for exacerbations and vaccination (see case 1). In this case, vaccination is not useful as the patient has hypogammaglobulinaemia. Normal investigation of additional causes of bronchiectasis may be equally limited in this case (e.g. *Aspergillus* precipitins).

Other investigations

Further investigation is required to clarify the abnormalities seen on the HRCT scan (nodularity, infiltrates), especially if they do not clear after treatment for the infection. Bronchoalveolar lavage is an important investigation to exclude atypical infection (e.g. fungi, non-tuberculous mycobacteria) and malignancy.

Progress

The patient underwent eradication therapy for *Pseudomonas* (oral ciprofloxacin and nebulized colomycin for 4 weeks) with subsequent negative sputum cultures. The CXR abnormalities persisted, and she continued to complain of shortness of breath and malaise. Bronchoalveolar lavage was conducted, showing no evidence of infection or malignancy, with increased numbers of lymphocytes and negative for microbiology including AFBs. A repeat CT scan 2 months later (not shown) showed increase in the infiltrate and nodularity.

Question

35h) What is the differential diagnosis for these persistent CT changes and how would you proceed?

Answer

35h) **What is the differential diagnosis for these persistent CT changes and how would you proceed?**

The differential diagnosis radiologically includes lymphoid interstitial pneumonia (LIP), primary lymphoma of the lung and non-tuberculous mycobacteria. The negative lavage makes non-tuberculous mycobacteria highly unlikely.

LIP is not bronchocentric in nature, and therefore transbronchial biopsies are unlikely to be helpful, and produce too small a sample to assess for lymphoma (transbronchial biopsies may be useful in this context as an aid to the diagnosis of atypical infection, but will not help to achieve one of the diagnoses above). An open lung biopsy is, therefore, reasonable, to enable firm diagnosis, treatment and prognostication.

Progress

She underwent open lung biopsy, histology of which showed an interstitial infiltrate of lymphocytes and plasma cells along the alveolar septae, with no evidence of clonality.

Questions

35i) What is the diagnosis?

35j) How would you manage this condition?

35k) What diseases is it associated with?

Answers

35i) **What is the diagnosis?**

The histology is consistent with a diagnosis of lymphoid interstitial. pneumonia (LIP). The disease is defined as a dense interstitial lymphoid infiltrate (including lymphocytes, plasma cells, histiocytes) with extensive infiltration of the alveolar septae. There are lymphoid follicles and lymphoid hyperplasia present within the pulmonary lymphatics and non-caseating granulomas may be seen.

Lymphoid interstitial pneumonia is an uncommon disease classified within the idiopathic interstitial pneumonias. It most commonly affects female patients in the fifth decade, and usually presents insidiously with increasing cough and breathlessness over a period of years. LIP is usually associated with another disease (see answer 35k).

◆ Radiological features. LIP may present in a wide variety of radiological patterns. Two main CXR patterns have been described: basal interstitial changes associated with air space shadowing, and diffuse airspace involvement associated with honeycombing. On CT, ground glass shadowing is usually seen and may be associated with peri-vascular honeycombing or cyst formation. Multi-focal nodularity +/– consolidation and reticulation may also be seen.

◆ Diagnosis is made on the basis of clinical suspicion (especially in the presence of associated disease states as below) plus histology. The radiological features of LIP may occur in many infective/inflammatory diseases, and therefore histological proof is usually sought. The main differential diagnosis (once infection has been excluded) is of pulmonary lymphoma, in which case a clonal population of lymphocytes is seen, and there may be evidence of tumour tracking along the lymphatics.

Whereas LIP was previously considered to be a pre-malignant condition that inevitably developed in to lymphoma, only a small number of cases have been shown to follow this pattern and the majority of cases should be considered to be non-malignant.

35j) **How would you manage this condition?**

Oral corticosteroids are the usual form of treatment, with radiological monitoring of response, although there are no trials on which to base practise in this rare disease. Authorities recommend a prednisolone dose of 0.75–1mg/kg bodyweight for 8 to 12 weeks initially, followed by an attempt to reduce dose. Cases may resolve spontaneously, although around one-third progress to diffuse lung fibrosis. In this case, steroid treatment resulted in a dramatic clinical and radiological improvement. Over the following 2-year period, high doses of steroids were required, however, and were associated with significant complications.

Prognosis and required length of therapy is unknown. In around one-third of patients, progression occurs associated with poor prognosis, resulting in death in a median of 20 months.

35k) **What diseases is it associated with?**

Associated conditions:

- Auto-immune conditions, e.g. rheumatoid arthritis, SLE, haemolytic anaemia, myasthenia, pernicious anaemia, thyroid disease
- Sjögren's syndrome (one-quarter of cases of LIP are reported to be associated with Sjögren's)
- Immunodeficiency—as seen here, e.g. in HIV, inherited conditions
- Drug-induced (captopril and phenytoin)
- Infections (e.g. Epstein Barr virus, pneumocystis pneumonia, hepatitis B).

Further reading

Demedts M, Costabel U (2002). ATS/ERS international multidisciplinary consensus classification of the idiopathic interstitial pneumonias. *Eur Respir J*; **19** (5): 794–796.

Swigris JJ, Berry GJ, Raffin TA, Kuschner WG (2002). Lymphoid interstitial pneumonia: a narrative review. *Chest*; **122** (6): 2150–2164.

Case 36

A 74-year-old woman was referred to the chest clinic with a 4-month history of malaise, cough, sputum production and an abnormal CXR. She had been treated with several courses of different antibiotics by her GP with some symptomatic response over that period. She had a past history of left breast carcinoma 20 years previously, treated with local resection and high-dose radiotherapy. The patient reported significant skin damage after radiotherapy, and CXRs from 15 years previously, reviewed in the clinic, showed evidence of early left-upper zone fibrosis and mild volume loss.

She was a life-long non-smoker with no other risk factors for respiratory disease. Her past medical history was otherwise unremarkable.

On examination, chest expansion was decreased on the left, and the trachea was deviated to the left. There were crackles, and areas of bronchial breathing within the left-upper zone, respiratory rate was 16, and oxygen saturation was 92% on room air. There was no clubbing or lymphadenopathy.

Investigations

- Mildly raised inflammatory markers (ESR 36mm/h, CRP 62mg/L)
- Normocytic anaemia (Hb = 9.8g/dL, MCV = 74fL).
- CXR in Fig. 36.1 and CT in Fig. 36.2.

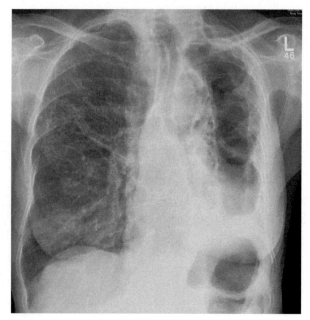

Fig. 36.1 CXR.

She proceeded to CT scanning of the chest, for which images of the right lung are shown only (Fig. 36.2).

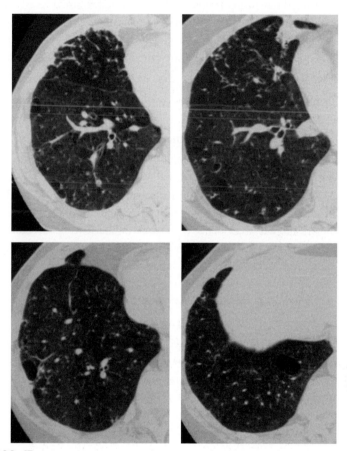

Fig. 36.2 CT scans.

Questions

36a) Describe the CXR (Fig. 36.1).

36b) Describe the chest CT findings (Fig. 36.2)

36c) Suggest a possible differential diagnosis for this presentation.

36d) What investigations would you arrange?

Answers

36a) **Describe the CXR (Fig. 36.1).**

The CXR shows volume loss in the left lung (raised hemidiaphragm, rib crowding, hilar displacement, ipsilateral tracheal shift) in association with areas of reticulation and linear atelectasis. In addition, a fluid level is apparent. Nodularity and subtle consolidation are seen within the right-upper lobe, with a raised horizontal fissure.

36b) **Describe the chest CT findings (Fig. 36.2)**

The CT images reveal ill-defined scattered nodules, peripheral consolidation and areas of emphysema.

36c) **Suggest a possible differential diagnosis for this presentation.**

The radiographic features are consistent with a chronic fibrotic reaction (volume loss and atelectasis), which may, in this case, be a result of the previous high-dose radiotherapy treatment. Alternative causes of a chronic fibrotic reaction would include previous chronic empyema and old tuberculosis. There is no evidence of fissural nodularity (e.g. sarcoidosis) or peripheral bilateral honeycombing (e.g. UIP). The clinical features (malaise, productive cough) are suggestive of a secondary infection and, given the presence of damaged areas of lung, a broad range of pathogens (including fungi) should be considered.

36d) **What investigations would you arrange?**

Suitable investigations would include sputum culture (induced sputum, if necessary) with bronchoscopy and bronchoalveolar lavage (BAL), if unable to obtain sputum. Acid-fast bacilli stains and culture and fungal culture should be requested.

Progress

A single sputum culture was undertaken, which revealed moderate amounts of acid-fast bacilli on ZN staining. She was, therefore, commenced on quadruple therapy (rifampicin, isoniazid, pyrazinamide and ethambutol) while microbiological sensitivities were awaited.

She was reviewed 2 months after commencing therapy and was changed to a two-drug regimen (rifampicin and isoniazid). One week later, final microbiological cultures from the sputum suggested mycobacteria avium complex (MAC).

Questions

36e) What is the diagnosis at this stage?

36f) What is the next investigation?

36g) How would you manage this patient?

Answers

36e) What is the diagnosis at this stage?

Although the clinical features are consistent with a diagnosis of non-tuberculous mycobacterial (NTM) pulmonary infection, MAC has only been isolated in one microbiological sample (sputum). This does not meet the criteria for diagnosis of NTM infection (see later), and further investigations are required.

36f) What is the next investigation?

Further microbiological samples are required to confirm the presence of an NTM to suggest a diagnosis of pulmonary infection (rather than airway colonisation). Bronchoscopy and bronchoalveolar lavage should be considered if sputum is not diagnostic. Other diagnoses (e.g. *Aspergillus*, carcinoma, tuberculosis) should be excluded.

36g) How would you manage this patient?

If MAC is the causative organism, the current antibiotic regimen is likely to be ineffective. However, treatment of NTM requires prolonged therapy with potential side-effects, and therefore the priority in this case is to firmly establish diagnosis. Four further sputum cultures (induced) were taken on two separate occasions, all of which consistently grew MAC.

Questions

36h) Describe the main features of NTM pulmonary disease.

36i) Describe the diagnostic criteria for NTM pulmonary disease.

36j) How would you manage such a patient?

Answers

36h) **Describe the main features of NTM pulmonary disease.**

- Definition of NTM. NTM are ubiquitous environmental organisms, which do not belong to the *Mycobacterium tuberculosis* complex or *Mycobacterium leprae*. Around 90% of disease due to NTM is pulmonary, with the remaining being superficial lymphadenitis (especially in children), skin or soft tissue infections, and disseminated disease in the immunocompromised.

- Mycobacterium avium complex (MAC). This term includes either *Mycobacterium avium* or *Mycobacterium intracellulare* (two species that are difficult to differentiate), and are the commonest NTM to cause pulmonary disease, most often in patients with pre-existing lung disease (e.g. fibrosis, COPD, bronchiectasis). Clinical features may be non-specific (cough, fatigue, weight loss, malaise). Disease is characterized by progressive pulmonary disease, usually in immunocompetent hosts. Three major clinical syndromes are described:

  - Disease presenting similarly to *Mycobacterium tuberculosis* with systemic illness, upper lobe infiltrates and cavities, most often in elderly male smokers with COPD. Extensive parenchymal damage is not uncommon as presentation is often late, as the disease is usually less aggressive than *Mycobacterium tuberculosis*.
  - MAC in an area of pre-existing bronchiectasis (any cause but often prior TB or cystic fibrosis)
  - Female non-smokers over 50 years old with no pre-existing lung condition, in association with interstitial shadowing (known as 'Lady Windermere syndrome').

  Associated systemic features may include bone marrow involvement (anaemia, neutropaenia), lymphadenopathy, hepatosplenomegaly, GI and liver involvement. Disseminated infection may occur in the immunocompromised.

- *Mycobacterium kansasii*. Presents in a manner similar to *M. tuberculosis*, with cavitation in the majority of cases and bilateral disease in 20%.

- Rapidly growing mycobacteria. These organisms grow in culture within 1 week and include *Mycobacterium fortuitum*, *Mycobacterium chelonae* and *Mycobacterium abscessus*. This most often occurs as disseminated disease in the immunocompromised, particularly in HIV positive patients.

36i) **Describe the diagnostic criteria for NTM pulmonary disease.**

Diagnostic criteria (American Thoracic Society 2007). Requires all of the following:

◆ Relevant symptoms

◆ Consistent radiological abnormalities

◆ Exclusion of other disease processes (e.g. fungal disease)

◆ Microbiological confirmation of disease rather than colonization. Regardless of smear positivity, this requires at least one of:

  • Two positive sputum cultures

  • Single positive bronchoalveolar lavage

  • Single biopsy (transbronchial or other) with consistent histology (granulomas) and positive culture

  • Single biopsy with consistent histology plus positive sputum culture

  • Positive culture from a privileged site (e.g. pleural effusion).

Clinical features:

◆ Often reflect the underlying disease (e.g. COPD, bronchiectasis)

◆ Pulmonary symptoms (cough/dyspnoea/haemoptysis)

◆ Systemic symptoms (malaise/fever/weight loss/lethargy).

Radiology:

◆ Variable according to type of NTM

◆ HRCT is more sensitive in detecting many of the radiographic features of NTM disease

◆ Think of NTM in cases of:

  • Multiple small nodules

  • Cavitatory disease

  • Multifocal bronchiectasis

  • Nodular infiltrates.

◆ Cavitatory disease:

  • 50% of MAC

  • 90% of *M. kansasii.*

◆ Nodules/bronchiectasis:

  • 50% of MAC

  • Most often seen in the right middle lobe.

36j) **How would you manage such a patient?**

Treatment principles:

◆ Single agent therapy is not recommended

◆ Sensitivities may be helpful in long treatment course, but *in vitro* may not reflect *in vivo* sensitivity

◆ There are no randomized trials of therapy in immunocompetent hosts

◆ Treatment is generally recommended until cultures have been repeatedly negative over a 1-year period and this usually involves at least 18–24 months treatment

◆ It is recommended that drug toxicity (hepatic, GI, haematological, renal, vision) is monitored once monthly due to long duration of therapy

◆ Newer evidence suggests that macrolides and quinolones may have a role (Jenkins *et al.* 2008)

Regimens (daily): triple therapy in all cases.

◆ Cavitatory MAC:
  - Clarithromycin 500–1000mg OR azithromycin 250mg and
  - Rifampicin 600mg or rifabutin 150–300mg and
  - Ethambutol 15mg/kg.

◆ Nodular MAC:
  - Clarithromycin 1000mg OR azithromycin 500mg and
  - Rifampicin 600mg or rifabutin 150–300mg and
  - Ethambutol 25mg/kg.

◆ *M. kansasii*:
  - Isoniazid 300mg and
  - Rifampicin 600mg and
  - Ethambutol 15mg/kg.

◆ Surgical options. Consider surgical resection in complicated cases where there is a combination of localized disease plus inability to tolerate drug regimens, or presence of resistant strains (e.g. culture positive after 6 months treatment).

Further reading

Jenkins PA, Campbell IA, Banks J, Gelder CM, Prescott RJ, Smith AP (2008). Clarithromycin *vs* ciprofloxacin as adjuncts to rifampicin and ethambutol in treating opportunist mycobacterial lung diseases and an assessment of *Mycobacterium vaccae* immunotherapy. *Thorax*; **63**: 627–634.

Zumla AI, Grange J (2002). Non-tuberculous mycobacterial pulmonary infections. *Clin Chest Med*; **23**: 369–376.

Case 37

A 45-year-old man with a 5-year history of COPD had become increasingly symptomatic in recent months, with frequent exacerbations and several admissions, receiving non-invasive ventilation on one occasion. Dyspnoea during activities (such as getting dressed) and poor exercise tolerance limited him to walking around the house only (6-min walk distance markedly reduced at 140m). He was an ex-smoker with a 40 pack-year history, and had suffered with asthma since childhood. He had a right-sided pneumothorax a year previously, which failed to resolve with chest drain insertion and attempted talc pleurodesis. A Heimlich flutter valve was therefore substituted for the underwater seal in order to allow him to go home until the pneumothorax resolved some months later.

He suffered from low mood, which he attributed to ill health due to being unable to work and difficulty looking after his children. He was on maximum inhaled therapy (steroids, a long acting beta agonist, and tiotropium), and required frequent courses of oral prednisolone and antibiotics. He had a squamous cell carcinoma removed from his cheek 6 months previously.

Investigations

Table 37.1 Pulmonary function tests

	Measured and (% predicted) values
BMI(kg/m^2)	30.2
FEV$_1$(L)	0.6 (15%)
FVC(L)	2.0 (43%)
FEV$_1$/FVC ratio	30%
FRC(L)	6.4 (186%)
RV(L)	4.9 (241%)
TLC(L)	8.5 (121%)
TL$_{CO}$(mM/min/kPa)	5.48 (51%)
K$_{CO}$(mM/min/kPa/L)	0.8 (53%)

Table 37.2 Arterial blood gases

pH	7.41
SaO$_2$ (%)	89
PaCO$_2$ (kPa)	7.3
PaO$_2$ (kPa)	7.1
BE (mM/L)	9.2
HCO$_3^-$ (mM/L)	31.6

Question

37a) Discuss interventions, other than inhaled medications, that should be considered for this man. Give criteria for their use.

Answer

37a) **Discuss interventions, other than inhaled medications, that should be considered for this man. Give criteria for their use.**

Severe COPD is a common condition, with a large symptom burden for the patient, significant health-resource implications and a high mortality. Management aims to:

- Reduce disease progression
- Minimize exacerbation frequency
- Ameliorate symptoms
- Increase coping strategies.

This man may be suitable for long-term oxygen therapy (LTOT)—oxygen supplementation for at least 15h a day. His single arterial blood gas fulfils the criteria for LTOT (PaO_2 <7.3 kPa, or <8.0 kPa in the presence of hypercapnia or cor pulmonale), and he would need a further blood gas taken, when stable, to verify this. Oxygen is supplemented at a flow rate sufficient to raise PaO_2 to >8kPa, without developing a rise in $PaCO_2$ and thus respiratory acidosis. It improves survival in selected patients with COPD and chronic hypoxia after at least 1 year of treatment, with those with greater degrees of hypoxia and cor pulmonale receiving most benefit.

He should be referred for pulmonary rehabilitation. This is of benefit for COPD patients who are dyspnoeic on walking but can manage at least 30m, and have an FEV_1 < 60% predicted. Pulmonary rehabilitation improves exercise tolerance and dyspnoea, is associated with reduced hospital stays and improvement in quality of life. A significant part of this course is exercise training, which patients are encouraged to continue long-term.

Ideally all patients with COPD should be offered nutritional assessment and help in optimizing of weight. The patient in this case is overweight, which will increase his work of breathing and oxygen requirements during exercise. This is better than being underweight, however, as this has an adverse impact on survival compared to those of normal or increased weight. Optimizing nutrition is particularly important during exacerbations, especially if oral intake is impaired due to use of non-invasive or invasive ventilatory support, and feeding via a nasogastric tube may need to be considered. This also applies to overweight patients, as a low albumin, phosphate or magnesium may have an adverse impact on recovery and weaning from ventilation.

This man could have a trial of low-dose opiates or benzodiazepines before activities that he knows make him breathless, such as getting dressed, with the aim of relieving dyspnoea and anxiety. Titrated in small doses they do not lead to worsening hypercapnia or premature death.

Non-invasive ventilation is of benefit during acute hypercapnic, acidotic exacerbations; however, there remains insufficient evidence to recommend long-term home use in COPD, even in the presence of a chronically raised $PaCO_2$.

Occasionally, in carefully selected cases, surgical treatment, such as lung volume reduction surgery, bullectomy or transplant can be considered, and these are discussed further below.

Given the poor prognosis of severe COPD, patients and their carers should be given the opportunity to discuss end-of-life wishes, including ITU admissions in the future.

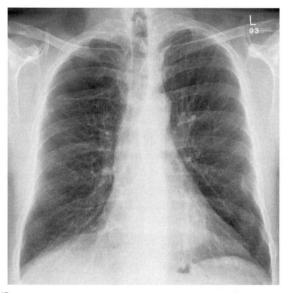

Fig. 37.1 CXR.

Questions

37b) Describe the features illustrated by the CXR (Fig. 37.1).

37c) What further imaging is required to decide whether a patient may benefit from lung transplantation?

Answers

37b) Describe the features illustrated by the CXR (Fig. 37.1).

The CXR shows hyperinflated lung fields. A large area of lucency is seen at the right apex, which is almost certainly related to a bulla, rather than a pneumothorax (supported by the concave inferior margin). Callus formation due to old rib fractures are seen at the left base.

37c) What further imaging is required to decide whether a patient may benefit from lung transplantation?

Further imaging required when considering lung transplantation. A CT-chest is required to examine the distribution of lung disease, and to exclude other factors that might contra-indicate transplant, such as a lung cancer. An echocardiogram and bone densitometry are also required, as a poor ejection fraction, or osteoporosis would make transplant surgery too high risk.

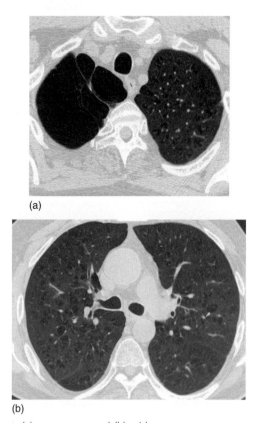

(a)

(b)

Fig. 37.2 CT chest. (a) upper zone and (b) mid zone.

Questions

37d) Describe the features illustrated by the CT-chest (Fig. 37.2a and b).

37e) Discuss the factors in this man's case that should be taken into account when deciding whether or not he should be considered for lung transplantation.

37f) How may survival in COPD be predicted?

Answers

37d) **Describe the features illustrated by the CT-chest (Fig. 37.2a and b).**

The upper zone CT chest slice (Fig. 37.2a) confirms right apical emphysematous changes with bullae formation. The mid zone CT chest slice (Fig. 37.2b) shows moderate centrilobar emphysema in both lung, and, although multiple slices are not shown, this was seen throughout the rest of the lung fields.

37e) **Discuss the factors in this man's case that should be taken into account when deciding whether or not he should be considered for lung transplantation.**

Factors to take into account when considering transplant referral. Surgical intervention is only appropriate for a small minority of patients with severe COPD due to the strict eligibility criteria and limited organ supply; however, it should still be considered. Lung transplantation in COPD may improve exercise tolerance and quality of life for carefully selected patients. However, deciding the optimal time of referral is challenging; many patients suffer for years with significant symptoms, making it difficult to identify patients with a high short-term mortality risk. The survival advantage of lung transplant in COPD (82% at 1 year, 49% at 5 years) compared to survival without transplant is not fully known. Selecting patients at the more severe end of the spectrum increases the probability that transplant will improve survival, so long as comorbidity does not increase operative risk unreasonably. The man in this case has a significant predicted mortality based on several criteria described in answer (37f), and therefore transplant should be considered.

Contraindications to transplant. This man has no absolute contraindications: he is not a current smoker, and, although an active malignancy within the previous 2 years is a contraindication, basal and squamous cell carcinoma of the skin are exceptions to this. Medical conditions, such as diabetes and hypertension, are relative contraindications only if they are not well controlled or have resulted in end-organ damage. Oral prednisolone is no longer a contraindication to transplant unless there is associated osteoporosis, though attempts should be made to minimize the dose, to less than 20mg/day at least. This man would need evaluation of his mental health and adherence to previous therapies, as poorly controlled psychoaffective disorders, often leading to poor adherence to therapy, are relative contraindications to transplant. Cyclomegalovirus is no longer a contraindication to transplantation, as infection can be prevented or controlled with ganciclovir.

One of the considerations for this man is his previous talc slurry pleurodesis. This would make any form of thoracic surgery longer and more difficult, although does not affect the eventual outcome; there is a higher risk of bleeding and greater inotropic requirement and, in lung volume reduction surgery, the risk of a prolonged air leak is increased. It is thought that prior abrasion pleurodesis may result in fewer surgical complications than talc slurry pleurodesis. In terms of other pleural procedures, a previous full pleurectomy would be an absolute contraindication to transplant.

37f) **How may survival in COPD be predicted?**

Predicting survival in severe COPD. Data from the National Emphysema Treatment Trial (NETT), suggested that patients with COPD and an FEV_1 <20% predicted, as does the man in this case, and have a median survival of 3 years. This study also found a TL_{CO} <20%, or homogenous disease on high-resolution computed tomography, to be predictive of poor prognosis.

The 'BODE' index takes more factors into account, and was specifically developed to help predict survival in COPD. It is based upon **B**ody mass index, the degree of airflow **O**bstruction (% predicted FEV_1), **D**yspnoea (modified Medical Research Council dyspnoea scale) and **E**xercise tolerance (6-min walk distance). The man in this case has a BODE index of 8, which would suggest a median survival of 3 years. He has also had a hospital admission with an exacerbation complicated by hypercapnia ($PaCO_2$ >6.0kPa); such patients have a median 2-year survival of only 50%.

Additional poor prognostic factors are pulmonary hypertension, hypoxaemia, hypercapnia multiple exacerbations, and a low haematocrit.

Question

37g) What factors would need to be taken into account, if considering referral for lung volume reduction surgery (LVRS), compared to transplant?

Answer

37g) **What factors would need to be taken into account, if considering referral for lung volume reduction surgery (LVRS), compared to transplant?**

The rationale of LVRS is to improve the mismatch between the size of the lungs and of the thoracic cavity by removing space-occupying, hyper-inflated, emphysematous areas of lung that contribute least to gas exchange. In the remaining lung, the hope is to improve elastic recoil and airways resistance by allowing it to expand. It is, therefore, of greatest benefit in patients with heterogenous disease. This is borne out by the Nation Emphysema Treatment Trial (NETT), in which LVRS led to an improvement in exercise capacity and quality of life in 'all comers', but only reduced mortality in patients with predominant upper-lobe disease.

The man in this case could, theoretically, be considered for LVRS as he has heterogenous disease, with marked bullous emphysema in his right-upper lobe. He could also, theoretically, be considered for bullectomy, as he has an isolated bulla occupying >30% of a hemithorax, with relatively underexpanded underlying lung. However, he has an FEV_1 <20% predicted, putting him at high mortality risk from surgery. Other factors (not relevant to this patient) making LVRS or bullectomy a higher risk than medical therapy alone, are TL_{CO} <20% predicted, homogeneous disease on CT scan, PaO_2 <6kPa, bronchiectasis with chronic sputum production, age >70 years old, pulmonary hypertension (peak systolic pulmonary arterial pressure of >50mmHg) and previous thoracic surgery.

Advantages of LVRS or bullectomy over transplant are that they are not constrained by a limited organ supply and, of particular relevance to the patient in this case, life-long immunosuppression is not required; the necessity of numerous essential regular medications is sometime difficult in patients with mental health problems. Studies on a bronchoscopic 'equivalent of LVRS', using endobronchial one-way valves, are currently underway, which may become an option for patients who are not fit enough for a major surgical procedure.

Further reading

Ambrosino N, Simonds A (2007). The clinical management in extremely severe COPD. *Respir Med*; **101**: 11613–11624.

Celli BR, Cote GG, Marin JM, Casanova C, Montes de Oca M, Mendez RA *et al.* (2004). The body-mass index, airflow obstruction, dyspnea, and exercise capacity index in chronic obstructive pulmonary disease. *N Engl J Med*; **350** (10): 1005–1012.

Glanville AR, Estenne M (2003). Indications, patient selection and timing of referral for lung transplantation. *Eur Respir J*; **22**: 845–852.

National Emphysema Treatment Trial Research Group (2003). Cost effectiveness of lung-volume reduction surgery for patients with severe emphysema. *New Engl J Med*; **348**: 2092–2102.

Patel N, DeCamp M, Criner GJ (2008). Lung transplant and lung volume reduction surgery versus transplantation in chronic obstructive pulmonary disease. *Proc Am Thorac Soc*; **5**: 447–453.

Sayeed RA, Waddell TK (2008). Lung volume reduction surgery. In: *Core Topics in Cardiothoracic Critical Care* (Klein A, Nashef SAM, eds) Cambridge University Press, chapter 52, pp. 392–396.

Case 38

A 67-year-old lady was referred with 6 months of progressive breathlessness on exertion. Her past medical history was of limited Wegener's granulomatosis, diagnosed 15 years previously, causing recurrent nasal and sinus disease and requiring frequent sinus irrigation. She had remained ANCA negative over recent years and was currently on no immunosuppressive treatment, but had been treated with steroids, cyclophosphamide and azathioprine shortly after diagnosis. On examination, resting SaO_2 was 97%, there were fairly harsh inspiratory and expiratory sounds (no frank stridor) and signs of previous Wegener's with collapsed nasal bridge. Full examination was otherwise normal.

Table 38.1 Pulmonary function tests

	Measured	% Predicted
PEFR(L/min)	140	41
FEV_1(L)	1.8	88
FVC(L)	3.0	120
FEV_1/FVC	61	
RV(L)	3.5	133
TLC(L)	5.5	114
VA(L)	4.1	86
TL_{CO}(mmol/min/kPa)	5.47	76
K_{CO}(mmol/min/kPa/L)	1.33	89

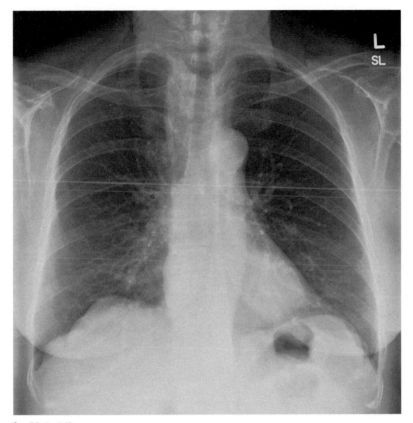

Fig. 38.1 CXR.

Questions

38a) What abnormality is suggested by the pulmonary function values (Table 38.1), and what further pulmonary function test would help?

38b) Interpret the CXR (Fig. 38.1).

38c) What two further investigations are required?

38d) What is the likely diagnosis?

Answers

38a) **What abnormality is suggested by the pulmonary function values (Table 38.1), and what further pulmonary function test would help?**

The pulmonary function (Table 38.1) shows mild airflow obstruction (and a small degree of air trapping). However, the peak flow is markedly reduced in comparison to the FEV_1. This suggests upper airway obstruction, and the Empey index—FEV_1(in ml)/PEFR(in L/min)—is 12.9. An Empey index of >10 is strongly suggestive of expiratory upper airway obstruction.

Suspicion of upper airway obstruction would be supported by examining a flow-volume loop (Fig. 38.2).

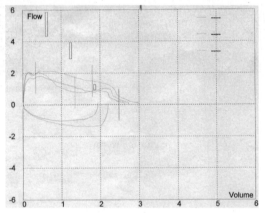

Fig. 38.2 Flow-volume loop. Expiration upwards, inspiration downwards, TLC far left of graph. Rectangles indicate normal range values, given the patient's VC.

38b) **Interpret the CXR (Fig. 38.1).**

The CXR shows diffuse widening of the right paratracheal soft tissues, and this has a well-defined slightly convex lateral margin. The right paratracheal stripe (tracheal wall outlined by air either side) is only preserved inferiorly (Fig. 38.3). The SVC up against the tracheal wall would not account for this abnormality, as it is never convex, and would not appear as dense as this, especially towards the apex (Fig. 38.3). There is no convincing significant tracheal indentation or narrowing (although this is just a PA projection and therefore elliptical narrowing with reduced antero-posterior tracheal dimensions may not be seen). Possible causes of this would be a goitre (although this should deviate the trachea), mediastinal fat or lipoma (although these would appear less dense).

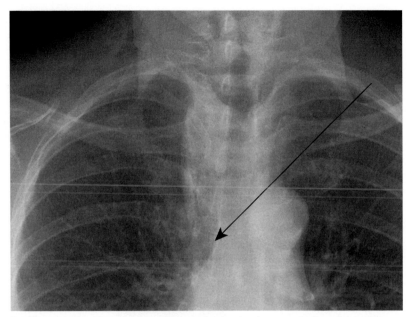

Fig. 38.3 CXR showing preserved paratracheal stripe lower end of trachea only (arrow).

38c) **What two further investigations are required?**

CT scan and bronchoscopy.

38d) **What is the likely diagnosis?**

Although the precise diagnosis of the clinical finding of upper airways obstruction is not clear at this point, a possibility is further upper airway involvement from Wegener's. The long history of nasal disease would raise the prior probability of this.

Further investigation

Bronchoscopy (Fig. 38.4) revealed marked narrowing of the trachea just below the vocal cords (to a diameter of approximately 5mm, in agreement with the CT scan). Distally, past the stenosis, the trachea appeared normal.

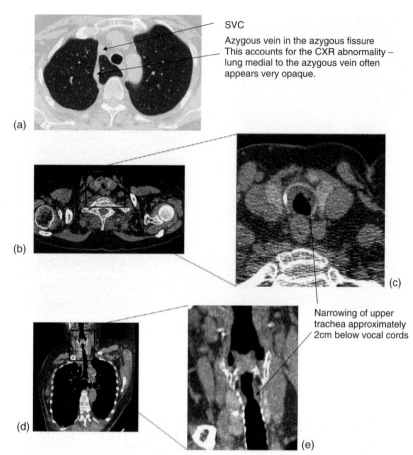

SVC

Azygous vein in the azygous fissure
This accounts for the CXR abnormality –
lung medial to the azygous vein often
appears very opaque.

(a)

(b)

(c)

Narrowing of upper
trachea approximately
2cm below vocal cords

(d)

(e)

Fig. 38.4 (a–c) Axial images from CT neck/thorax. (d,e) Coronal reconstruction showing narrowing of upper trachea.

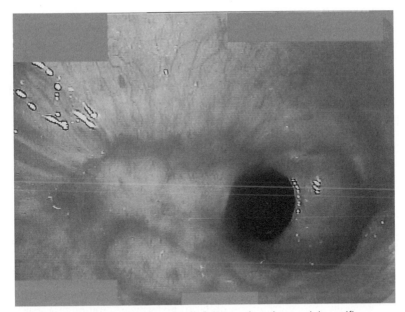

Fig. 38.5 Bronchoscopic view from level of the vocal cords, remaining orifice approximately 10% of normal tracheal cross-sectional area.

Questions

38e) What is the diagnosis?

38f) How does the flow volume loop vary with different causes of upper airflow obstruction?

38g) How would you manage this patient?

Answers

38e) **What is the diagnosis?**

Upper airway Wegener's granulomatosis causing post-inflammatory scarring and fibrosis in the trachea and a characteristic flow volume loop of fixed upper airflow obstruction.

38f) **How does the flow volume loop vary with different causes of upper airflow obstruction?**

The appearance of the flow volume loop (FVL) in upper airflow obstruction depends on whether the level of obstruction is intra or extrathoracic, or is fixed or variable.

In general, about half of the trachea is intrathoracic, and half extrathoracic. The upper extrathoracic part of the trachea is narrowed in inspiration as luminal pressure is subatmospheric. It will then dilate in expiration as luminal pressure exceeds that of its surroundings as intrathoracic pressure rises. Consequently, fleshy tumours in the upper trachea will generally cause more airflow obstruction during inspiration than expiration, and hence inspiratory stridor. In the lower trachea, in inspiration, the intraluminal pressure is higher than the surrounding negative intrathoracic pressure and the trachea dilates. In expiration, the lower trachea is compressed by surrounding positive intrathoracic pressure and the trachea is compressed. Therefore, with tumours in the lower trachea, stridor may be less immediately obvious as there will be more airflow obstruction in expiration than inspiration.

Clearly there may be mixed effects from tumours with more extensive upper airway involvement. The degree of differential impairment to the inspiratory or expiratory flow will also depend on the degree to which the obstruction is fixed. A more fleshy tumour in the upper trachea would be more likely to cause the effects above, as the obstructing elements are blown open in expiration. A more fibrotic or extensive submucosal tumour infiltration will cause similar levels of inspiratory and expiratory flow limitation. Typical FVL appearances would be:

- Variable extra-thoracic upper airway obstruction (e.g. vocal cord dysfunction—see case 29): relatively normal expiratory limb, flattening of inspiratory limb
- Variable intra-thoracic airway obstruction: relatively normal or slight impairment of inspiratory limb, flattening of expiratory limb
- Fixed upper airway obstruction: flattening of both inspiratory and expiratory limbs, so called 'square box' FVL.

38g) **How would you manage this patient?**

The treatment options are laser resection, tracheal dilatation or stenting with a decision made on an individual basis. In one series of 30 patients with endobronchial involvement by Wegener's (Daum *et al.* 1995), five had subglottic stenosis and four had tracheal or bronchial stenosis with other abnormalities including ulcerating tracheobronchitis. Three of these patients underwent dilatation and one had removal of granulation tissue by YAG laser, but symptoms had recurred in three of these four patients within 10 months. Three other patients underwent silastic stent insertion, which provided continued symptom relief over up to 33 months follow-up. In another series (Utzig *et al.* 2002) of eight patients with tracheal stenosis and five with subglottic stenosis who all underwent tracheal multiple tracheal dilatations, only one required stenting.

Our patient underwent dilatation of her subglottic stenosis with a good symptomatic result and has remained well since.

Further reading

Hetzel MR (2003). Diseases of the upper airway. In: Gibson GJ, Geddes DM, Costabel U, Sterk PJ, Corrin B. (eds) *Respiratory Medicine* (3rd edn). Saunders, London, chapter 44, pp. 1048–67.

Chapman S, Robinson G, Stradling JR, West S (2005). Lung function testing. In:*Oxford Handbook of Respiratory Medicine*. OUP, Oxford, Appendix 1, pp. 706–707.

Daum TE, Specks U, Colby TV, Edell ES, Brutinel MW, Prakash UB *et al.* (1995). Tracheobronchial involvement in Wegener's granulomatosis. *Am J Respir Crit Care Med*; **151** (2): 522–526.

Utzig MJ, Warzelhan J, Wertzel H, Berwanger I, Hasse J (2002). Role of thoracic surgery and interventional bronchoscopy in Wegener's granulomatosis. *Ann Thorac Surg*; **74**: 1948–1952.

Case 39

A 26-year-old man presented to the dermatologists with a 5-month history of a painless and non-itchy infiltrate in the red areas of a forearm tattoo. In addition, he noticed some small lumps that appeared on the elbow and outer arm above the tattoo. He had noticed some mild arthralgia over the last 3 months. There was no relevant past medical history, except that 2 years previously, the red areas in the tattoo had become raised but this had settled after a few weeks.

Patch-testing to various dyes used in tattoos was negative. He was given Tacrolimus cream on the assumption it was an allergic reaction to the red dye with no therapeutic effect. Some routine tests were performed.

Investigations

- FBC, U&Es and liver function tests were all normal
- Lung function, FEV$_1$/VC, 4.3/6.1(L), ratio 70%
- CXR in Fig. 39.1.

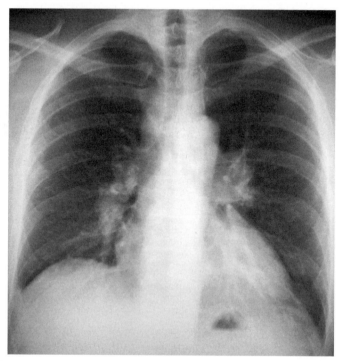

Fig. 39.1 CXR.

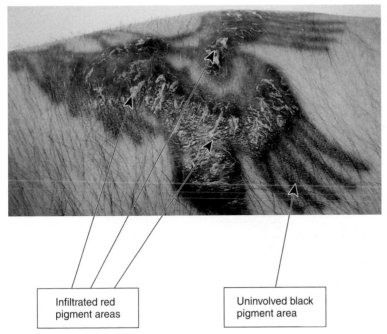

Infiltrated red
pigment areas

Uninvolved black
pigment area

Fig. 39.2 Skin tattoo (eagle).

Questions

39a) What does the CXR (Fig. 39.1) show?

39b) What is the likely diagnosis?

39c) What investigations would you do next?

39d) What treatment would you offer?

39e) Is the slightly low FEV_1/VC ratio compatible with the diagnosis?

Answers

39a) **What does the CXR (Fig. 39.1) show?**

The CXR (Figs. 39.1 and 39.3) shows bilateral hilar node enlargement and azygos node enlargement.

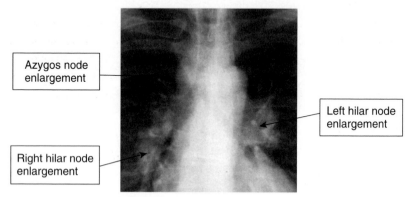

Azygos node enlargement

Left hilar node enlargement

Right hilar node enlargement

Fig. 39.3 Hilar area of CXR.

39b) **What is the likely diagnosis?**

The likely diagnosis is sarcoidosis. Infiltration with sarcoid granuloma of scars and tattoos is well recognized, and has been described particularly where there is red pigment, but also with navy blue and black pigments. One assumes the infiltration 2 years previously was the start of his sarcoidosis. Other causes of nodal enlargement would have to be considered in the absence of this pointer.

39c) **What investigations would you do next?**

Biopsy of the skin lesion showed typical non-caseating granuloma. A high-resolution CT scan of the chest might show typical micronodules in a subpleural, fissural and broncho-vascular distribution, and would have been useful if the diagnosis had not already been secure; but such a typical radiological pattern is not always present.

39d) **What treatment would you offer?**

Treatment would consist of steroid cream to the tattoo, ibuprofen and paracetamol for the arthralgia.

39e) **Is the slightly low FEV$_1$/VC ratio compatible with the diagnosis?**

The slightly low FEV$_1$/VC ratio may be due to the sarcoidosis, as there can be small airways obstruction, thought to be due to granulomatous involvement of small airways, usually, but not exclusively, when there is visible infiltration on the CXR. It can occur without a fall in compliance and VC (that would suggest an additional interstitial component), and may be evident on HRCT scanning as expiratory air trapping.

Progress

Symptoms resolved with simple treatments. Eight months later, dyspnoea and the tattoo infiltration returned. A repeat CXR was arranged and the radiologist organized an HRCT scan of the lungs. Before this appointment, the patient went on a beach holiday to Weymouth for 2 weeks. He became lethargic, with polyuria and thirst, and was admitted as an emergency on his return.

Investigations

- Urea 15mmol/L, Creatinine 411μmol/L, K$^+$ 5.3mmol/L
- See also Figs 39.4 and 39.5.

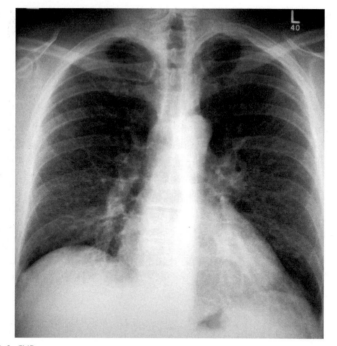

Fig. 39.4 CXR

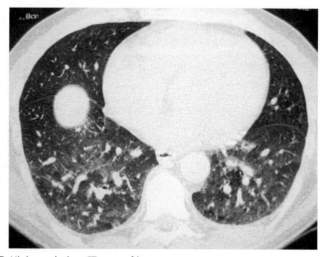

Fig. 39.5 High resolution CT scan of lungs.

Questions

39f) What do the CXR (Fig. 39.4) and HRCT (Fig. 39.5) show?

39g) What has happened?

39h) What test would you urgently order next?

39i) What is the relevance of the beach holiday?

39j) What is the treatment?

Answers

39f) **What do the CXR (Fig. 39.4) and HRCT (Fig. 39.5) show?**

The CXR now shows subtle infiltration with multiple small soft nodules, but the hilar have become essentially normal.

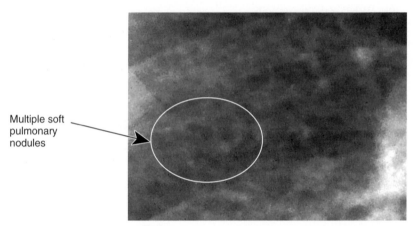

Multiple soft pulmonary nodules

Fig. 39.6 Magnified area of CXR.

The HRCT shows a diffuse nodular pulmonary infiltrate with some interlobar thickening compatible with, but not totally diagnostic of, sarcoidosis. There is no fissural nodularity, for example.

39g) **What has happened?**

He has developed renal failure due to several possible complications of sarcoidosis. Hypercalcaemia/hypercalcuria can damage the kidney slowly (though nephrocalcinosis) or acutely. About 40% of patients with sarcoidosis have hypercalciuria, but only about 15% develop hypercalcaemia. Hypercalcaemia also reduces responsiveness to ADH, producing polyuria and encouraging dehydration with pre-renal failure. A granulomatous nephritis can damage tubular function but is a rare cause of significant renal impairment.

39h) **What test would you urgently order next?**

A plasma calcium is required and was 3.32mmol/L on the day of admission. Activated macrophages in granuloma convert 25-hydroxyvitamin D into calcitriol $(1,25(OH)_2D_3)$, the most active version of vitamin D, thus resulting in increased absorption of calcium from the gut, and resorption from bone. This can occur in any granulomatous disease, not just sarcoidosis.

39i) **What is the relevance of the beach holiday?**

Sunlight from his beach holiday further increased the conversion of vitamin D to, ultimately, the active form, calcitriol, thus exacerbating the hypercalcaemia.

39j) **What is the treatment?**

Treatment is required with prednisolone (1mg/kg) and as generous intravenous fluids as the renal failure will allow. If hypercalcaemia alone is the reason for the renal failure, it will respond quickly. If dominantly nephrocalcinosis or a nephritis, the response is slower; failure to achieve normal renal function is associated with renal scarring. Further short-term calcium suppression can be obtained with pamidronate, if required. Long-term control of hypercalcaemia requires sun avoidance, a low calcium diet, low-dose steroids or hydroxychloroquine (via suppression of granuloma activity).

Progress

The hypercalcaemia resolved within 10 days, and the renal failure took nearly 4 months to fully resolve. Following a total of 7 months of steroids, these problems have not returned.

Case 40

A 44-year-old man was referred for evaluation following three episodes of small-volume haemoptysis (blood streaking of sputum only) in association with cough and purulent sputum production. His symptoms had resolved and he reported no further haemoptysis in the month prior to out-patient review. However, he did mention intermittent epistaxis for 'many years'.

He was a current smoker of 40 cigarettes a day (45 pack years).

On examination, he had multiple telangiectases on his lips and tongue. He was not anaemic or cyanosed, but his peripheral oxygen saturation was 91% on room air whilst sitting. His oxygen saturation rose to 95% when supine (SaO$_2$ 88% standing). His chest was clear.

His CXR (Fig. 40.1) and full pulmonary function testing, including transfer factor and diffusion capacity, were normal.

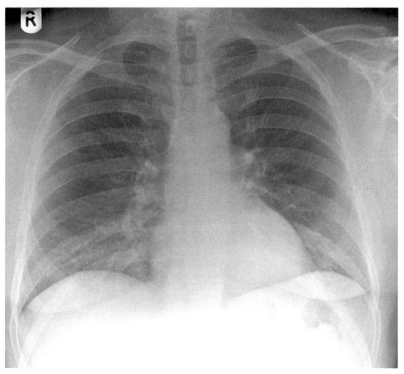

Fig. 40.1 CXR

Questions

40a) What is the likely diagnosis?

40b) What investigation would you do next?

Answers

40a) What is the likely diagnosis?

The history of epistaxis and physical findings of mucocutaneous tel-angiectasia suggest a diagnosis of hereditary haemorrhagic telangiectasia (HHT). Orthodeoxia (fall in arterial oxygen levels when upright) suggests associated pulmonary arteriovenous malformations (PAVM)—shunting and consequent desaturation are accentuated when upright due to an increased blood flow (with gravity) through, predominantly basally situated, AVM.

NB: a normal CXR does not exclude the diagnosis; clinically important PAVMs are often below the resolution of CXR.

40b) What investigation would you do next?

Contrast-enhanced thoracic CT is an appropriate next investigation. Contrast is not always needed, depending on institutional expertise. CT identifies PAVM and whether they are amenable to embolization. Additional lesions elsewhere in the lungs can be identified. Some centres would use contrast echocardiography if there was no clinical evidence of shunting present. Pulmonary angiography should usually be reserved for patients being considered for embolization.

Progress

On directed questioning, the patient reported that both his father and daughter also suffered with frequent epistaxis.

A CT pulmonary angiography was performed (Fig. 40.2) and demonstrated arteriovenous malformations anteriorly within the right-upper lobe (with a leading vessel identified, Fig. 40.2a) and in the postero-lateral segment of the right-lower lobe (arrowed, Fig. 40.2b). Elsewhere, multiple tiny AVMs were also identified.

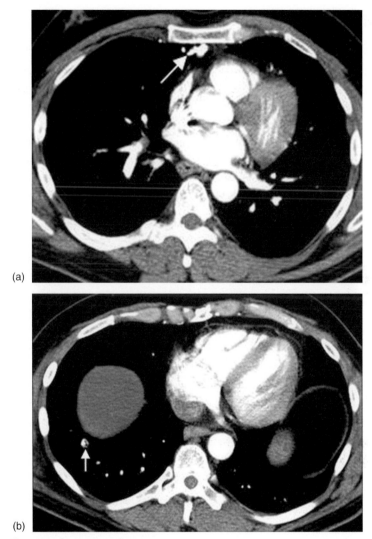

(a)

(b)

Fig. 40.2 CT pulmonary angiogram.

Question

40c) What would you do next to assess the clinical significance of the PAVM?

Answer

40c) **What would you do next to assess the clinical significance of the PAVM?**

All PAVMs are significant due to arterial hypoxaemia and potential paradoxical embolic stroke (Shovlin *et al.* 2008). The degree of right-to-left shunting, as the shunt fraction, can be measured.

Clinically significant PAVMs increase the fraction of cardiac output that bypasses the pulmonary capillary bed. In normal subjects, the intrapulmonary shunt is <2.5% of cardiac output and is mainly composed of left ventricular muscle venous blood draining directly into the left ventricle.

Progress

Radionuclide perfusion lung scanning was performed and an estimated shunt fraction of 12% calculated.

Questions

40d) How is the shunt fraction calculated via perfusion lung scanning?

40e) What other methods of shunt quantification may be used?

40f) What other tests could be used to detect PAVM?

40g) What are the complications of PAVM?

40h) What therapeutic options are there for this patient?

Answers

40d) How is the shunt fraction calculated via perfusion lung scanning?

The shunt fraction can be calculated in normal subjects by administration of intravenous ^{99m}Tc-labelled albumin macroaggregates, which are normally fully filtered by the pulmonary capillary bed. PAVMs allow their passage through the lungs, and thus their detection in other organs (e.g. kidneys and brain). Calculation of the shunt fraction is performed following differential radionuclide scanning over the lungs and right kidney (presumed to receive 10% of the cardiac output):

$$\text{Shunt fraction}(\%) = \left(\frac{\text{Right kidney counts} \times \text{correction factor} \times 10}{\text{Total counts injected}} \right) \times 100$$

The shunt fraction is raised in 90% or more of patients with PAVM.

40e) What other methods of shunt quantification may be used?

Other methods of quantification include the 100% oxygen method:

- Oxygen saturation and PaO_2 are measured after breathing 100% oxygen for 15–20min. A mouthpiece in combination with a nose-clip is much better than close fitting masks, or a non-rebreather system, as they tend to leak and not deliver 100% O_2. Administration of less than 100% will over-estimate the shunt fraction by lowering the P_AO_2.
- The shunt can be <u>accurately</u> calculated only if the mixed venous oxygen levels are known.

Fractional shunt = (pulmonary capillary O_2 content−arterial O_2 content)/ (pulmonary capillary O_2 content-mixed venous O_2 content)

or more commonly written

$$\text{Qshunt} \div \text{Qtotal} = (CAO_2 - CaO_2) \div (CAO_2 - C\bar{v}O_2)$$

where Q = blood flow, C = O_2 content, A = pulmonary capillary, a = arterial and $\bar{v}$ = mixed venous.

- However, an approximation can be made making various assumptions. If (i) the arterial oxygen saturation is 99 or 100% while breathing 100% oxygen (or PaO_2 > 25kPa),(ii) the Hb is 12–16g/dL, (iii) oxygen consumption/cardiac output normal, and (iv) the $PaCO_2$ is about 5.3 ± 0.5kPa, then the following very simplified equation can be used.

% shunt = 34−($PaO_2 \times 0.38$)

PaO_2 measured in kPa.

For example, if there is no shunt, then the arterial PaO_2 should be about 85kPa, if it were 60kPa, then $34 - (60 \times 0.38) = 11\%$ shunt.

- <10% shunt is probably normal (i.e. the PaO_2 on 100%O_2 is > 60kPa)

- 10–20% is abnormal, but not usually symptomatic (i.e PaO_2 on 100% O_2 is 35–60kPa).

- >20% is significant and usually symptomatic (i.e. PaO_2 on 100% O_2 is <35kPa).

40f) **What other tests could be used to detect PAVM?**

Other investigations used to evaluate intrapulmonary shunts include:

- Contrast echocardiography: involves injection of agitated saline (to introduce bubbles) into a peripheral vein whilst imaging the atria. In normal subjects the bubbles appear first in the right atrium, and then are trapped and dissipate in the pulmonary circulation. In patients with an intra-cardiac shunt, the bubbles are seen in the right atrium and within 1 cardiac cycle, in the left atrium. With PAVMs, after a delay of 3 to 8 cardiac cycles (2–5 seconds) contrast bubbles are seen in the left atrium.

- Contrast enhanced computed tomography: may be more sensitive than angiography in detection of PAVMs, although less able to determine the exact angioarchitecture.

- Pulmonary angiography: digital subtraction, or conventional, angiography is used (there are no existing comparison studies) and remain the gold standard. Pulmonary angiography is vital for treatment planning.

40g) **What are the complications of PAVM?**

Between 15 and 33% of patients with HHT have PAVMs (which originate from the pulmonary rather than bronchial arteries). Long-term complications include:

- Neurological
  - Stroke
  - Transient ischaemic attack (TIA)
  - Cerebral abscess
  - Seizure
  - Migraine.

These arise as a result of emboli reaching the cerebral circulation, bypassing the normal filtering system of the pulmonary capillaries, due to the right-to-left shunt, and may be the presenting feature of a PAVM. Strokes and abscesses are usually seen with feeding arteries >3mm in diameter.

More than two-thirds of cerebral phenomena seen in HHT arise due to emboli via PAVMs (the remainder due to additional cerebral AVMs, sometimes seen in HHT).

- ◆ Respiratory
  - Massive haemoptysis (rupture of a parenchymal PAVM or endo-bronchial telangiectasia)
  - Haemothorax (rupture of a subpleural PAVM).

Symptoms may develop or worsen during pregnancy as a consequence of an increased blood volume and cardiac output.

- ◆ Pulmonary hypertension—rare but may be related to defects in activin receptor-like kinase-1 (ALK-1), the product of one of the recognized underlying genetic mutations in HHT (HHT type 2).
- ◆ Other
  - Anaemia
  - Polycythaemia
  - Heart failure
  - Infective endocarditis.

40h) **What therapeutic options are there for this patient?**

Although the natural history of untreated PAVMs is unknown, approximately ¼ enlarge with time. Morbidity rates of up to 50% have been reported in patients with untreated PAVMs, compared to 3% of those following intervention. Treatment aims to prevent complications, particularly neurological, minimize progressive hypoxia and its sequelae, and reduce the incidence of high-output cardiac failure.

Current recommendations advise treatment of all symptomatic PAVMs and of those with feeding vessels ≥3mm.

Options include:

1. *Embolization therapy (embolotherapy)*: i.e. angiographic occlusion of the feeding arteries using steel coils or detachable balloons. This is the favoured initial therapeutic choice, particularly in patients not suitable for surgery, and those with multiple PAVMs (which can be embolized in a single session).

   Self-limiting pleuritic chest pain is the most common short-term complication (5–13%). Longer term stroke and/or cerebral abscess still occur in 2%, new PAVMs may develop and recanalization of treated PAVMs is seen in 1–10%. The development of pulmonary hypertension as a consequence of embolization (iatrogenic blockade of the low resistance AVMs), might be predicted, however, a recent study (Shovlin *et al.* 2008), did not show any significant increase in pulmonary artery pressures after embolization in 40 patients with HHT. The authors excluded patients with known advanced pulmonary hypertension for whom avoidance of PAVM embolization is currently recommended.

2. *Surgery*. Options include local excision, segmental or lobar resection and PAVM ligation. However, due to the morbidity associated with a general anaesthetic and thoracotomy, embolotherapy is preferred and surgery limited to those with allergy to contrast, or rarely PAVMs not amenable to embolization.

Long-term follow-up. The risk of growth of undetected PAVMs, and recanalization of embolized PAVMs, makes regular follow-up (clinical review and thoracic CT) prudent. Antibiotic prophylaxis is recommended, in those with treated or untreated PAVMs, prior to an invasive procedure, to reduce the risk of infection (via loss of the filtration afforded by the lung) such as cerebral abscess and infective endocarditis.

Screening of family members of those with HHT-related PAVMs is recommended, as the prevalence in relatives is approximately 35%. A thorough history, physical examination (with assessment for orthodeoxia using oximetry), CXR, 100% oxygen study and contrast echocardiogram are recommended screening tools in some centres.

Women with HHT should also be screened before pregnancy, as there is an increased rate of haemothorax and haemoptysis in the last half of pregnancy.

Progress

This patient was referred for formal pulmonary angiography and embolotherapy was subsequently performed with good effect.

Further reading

Gossage JR, Kani G (1998). Pulmonary arteriovenous malformations: a state of the art review. *Am J Respir Crit Care Med*; **158**: 643–661.

Shovlin CL, Jackson JE, Bamford KB, Jenkins IH, Benjamin AR, Ramadan H *et al.* (2008). Primary determinants of ischaemic stroke/brain abscess risks are independent of severity of pulmonary arteriovenous malformations in hereditary haemorrhagic telangiectasia. *Thorax*; **63**: 259–266.

Case 41

An 80-year-old woman was admitted to A&E with breathlessness. She had initially presented to her GP with a dry cough, and was diagnosed with a viral upper respiratory tract infection. Over the following three weeks she experienced progressive shortness of breath on exertion, and at presentation was breathless at rest. She denied sputum production, fevers and any constitutional symptoms.

Her past medical history included rheumatoid arthritis, which had been diagnosed 5 years previously. Her joint disease had been difficult to control on a combination of prednisolone 10mg once a day and methotrexate 15mg once weekly (with folate supplementation), and she had started anti-TNFa therapy three months ago with a reasonable response, enabling a decrease in her other therapy. There was no other relevant past medical history.

On examination she was tachypnoeic (35/min), afebrile and hypoxic (SaO_2 at rest 81% on room air). Investigations performed 3 weeks previously were compared to her admission investigations.

Investigations

Blood tests:

- This admission:
  - Hb, 8.8g/dL
  - WCC, 12.4×10^9/L (neutrophilia)
  - Platelets, 602×10^9/L
  - Urea and electrolytes normal
  - CRP >160mg/L.
- 3 weeks previously:
  - Hb, 9.5g/dL
  - WCC, 9.68×10^9/L
  - Platelets, 395×10^9/L
  - Urea and electrolytes normal
  - CRP = 35mg/L.
- Arterial blood gases (on air):
  - pH, 7.47
  - PaO_2, 6.2kPa
  - $PaCO_2$, 4.1kPa

- SaO_2, 81%
- Base excess, −0.8mM/L
- Bicarbonate, −24mM/L.
- See also Fig. 41.1.

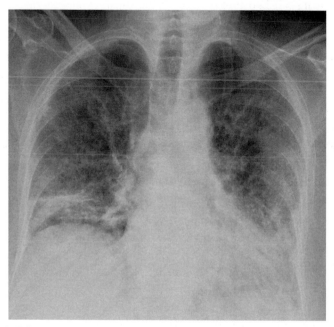

Fig. 41.1 CXR.

Questions

41a) Interpret the blood gas findings in this case.

41b) Describe the CXR findings (Fig. 41.1).

41c) What is the differential diagnosis and what is the most likely diagnosis. Why?

41d) Describe two key initial investigations and their rationale.

Answers

41a) **Interpret the blood gas findings in this case.**

The arterial blood gases show type I respiratory failure. The alveolar-arterial gradient (see case 12 for formula) is ~8kPa (normal 2–3)—this implies a substantial V/Q mismatch.

41b) **Describe the CXR findings (Fig. 41.1).**

The CXR shows:

- Bilateral volume loss
- Diffuse reticular opacification with a basal and peripheral predominance
- Opacification in the right-lower zone, which could be areas of atelectasis or consolidation.

41c) **What is the differential diagnosis and what is the most likely diagnosis. Why?**

The differential diagnosis here is one of multifocal, bilateral lung infiltrates in the context of rheumatoid arthritis. It includes:

1. Rheumatoid associated interstitial lung disease (RA-ILD). RA-ILD is the most common manifestation of rheumatoid lung disease. Radiologically, clinically and histologically, RA-ILD is similar to the idiopathic interstitial pneumonias, with usual interstitial pneumonitis (UIP), non-specific interstitial pneumonitis (NSIP) and cryptogenic organizing pneumonia (COP) the most common seen in rheumatoid. In this case, the bilateral volume loss and zonal distribution is in favour of UIP, whereas the relatively short history and aggressive progress is against this. UIP does not explain the right basal consolidation, whereas COP could cause this. However, COP is typically associated with bilateral infiltrates (as opposed to reticulation as seen here) and preserved lung volumes on CXR.

2. Drug induced lung disease. Pulmonary effects can result from a host of medication for the treatment of RA. Agents to consider are:

   - Methotrexate. Although infective complications are reported in patients treated with methotrexate (including PCP and fungal pneumonias), the most common pulmonary manifestation is acute pneumonitis (0.3 and 11.6% of patients). It is more common in those with underlying lung disease (including RA-ILD). It usually occurs within 2 years of starting therapy, but may occur after cessation of treatment. Diabetes, increased age and low albumin are all risk factors for acute pneumonitis. The clinical presentation is typically acute or subacute (weeks), and radiologically bilateral interstitial infiltrates or a combination of interstitial infiltrates and consolidation (as seen here) may occur.

- Corticosteroids. RA patients taking steroids are at greater risk of pneumonia requiring hospitalization. Taking prednisolone at ≥10mg per day for a month is a small but significant risk factor for PCP.

- Anti-TNFa therapy. All anti-TNFa and other biologic therapies for RA (e.g. B cell depletors, anti-IL1 therapy) have been associated with increased risk of pulmonary infections. The commonest is an association with bacterial pneumonia. There is also a well-known risk of the development of active pulmonary tuberculosis after initiation of anti-TNFa therapies, and screening is recommended prior to beginning such therapy (see British Thoracic Society website in Further reading). More recently, the use of anti-TNFa therapy has been associated with exacerbations and an increased risk of mortality (see Ostor *et al*), although further evidence is needed.

In this case, the clinical history and radiographic appearances make TB or other pulmonary infection alone unlikely. The time course of disease is very fast for RA-ILD alone. However, we are not given information on the patient's prior respiratory status (and she is quite likely to have been limited by joint disease therefore a history of exercise tolerance may be uninformative of her respiratory reserve) or exactly which drugs are being taken (i.e. is she still on methotrexate?). The two most likely possibilities are methotrexate induced pnuemonitis or undiagnosed and asymptomatic RA-ILD (most likely UIP) with intercurrent infection.

41d) **Describe two key initial investigations and their rationale.**

Important investigations include:

- Pulmonary function tests—these may aid in the diagnosis of RA-ILD (restrictive PFTs, small lung volumes, decreased TL_{CO}) or suggest COP (preserved volumes on CXR, decreased K_{CO}). However, this patient may be too compromised to perform anything except simple spirometry

- HRCT chest—this would enable assessment of the zonal predominance of the infiltrates (basal and subpleural implying UIP), the relative presence of ground glass and reticulation (NSIP or methotrexate pneumonitis versus UIP), consolidation (COP, intercurrent infection, PCP) and lobar involvement (pneumonia)

♦ Bronchoscopy, +/– lavage, +/– transbronchial biopsy. Exclusion of infection (lavage) before consideration of the other diagnoses is key, especially if the HRCT is not definitively RA-ILD and, as in this case, the history is short. Transbronchial biopsy may be useful in the diagnosis of COP, and provides a modest increase in diagnostic yield for PCP (around 10%)—however, it is unlikely that this patient would tolerate a pneumothorax.

♦ Consideration should be given to open lung biopsy if there is real diagnostic uncertainty after the above tests.

Progress

The patient was commenced on broad-spectrum antibiotic therapy, oxygen and thrombo-embolism prophylaxis and HRCT was performed (Fig. 41.2).

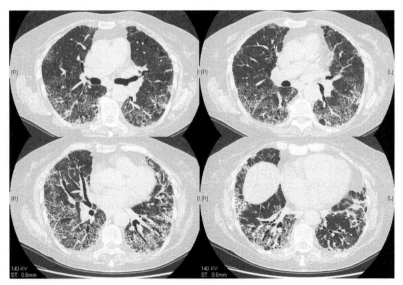

Fig. 41.2 HRCT chest.

Questions

41e) Describe the HRCT findings.

41f) What is the most likely diagnosis and what treatment would you consider?

Answers

41e) **Describe the HRCT findings.**

There is widespread ground glass opacification, with a peripheral, subpleural predominance (Fig. 41.3). On the basal cuts, there is coarse reticulation with areas of traction bronchiectasis (see Fig. 41.3).

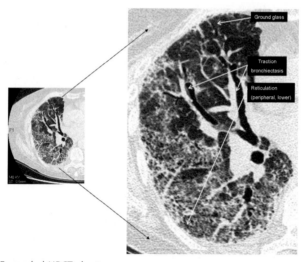

Fig. 41.3 Expanded HRCT chest.

41f) **What is the most likely diagnosis and what treatment would you consider?**

The HRCT is suggestive of RA-ILD with coarse reticulation and traction dilatation of airways (or 'bronchiectasis'; implying a chronic fibrotic process, e.g. UIP). The ground glass opacity may represent an additional pathology (e.g. drug-induced lung disease, infection, inflammation such as NSIP) or established fibrosis, which is beyond the resolution of the CT scanner. Given the acute deterioration in the patient, the putative diagnosis of RA-ILD (UIP) in association with methotrexate induced pneumonitis was made.

Treatment of methotrexate induced pneumonitis:

- Immediate cessation of methotrexate
- Patients will usually respond to this alone, but high-dose oral steroids are recommended to speed recovery if patients are acutely unwell (as here)

- In general, methotrexate should be avoided in the future (although if no other therapeutic options exist, slow re-introduction and careful monitoring of pulmonary function and CXR may be considered).

Treatment of RA-ILD (UIP):

- There are no large studies addressing the management of patients with RA-ILD and treatment is based on the associated idiopathic interstitial pneumonia (i.e. UIP).
- NSIP and COP are, therefore, treated with oral steroids, as per the treatment of non-RA entities.
- The treatment of RA-UIP is more controversial. There are many case reports of successful treatment with a variety of anti-RA drugs, but all of these are associated with possible significant pulmonary toxicity.
- One study has suggested that anti-TNFα therapy may slow progression of RA-ILD, but another has reported severe respiratory failure with this treatment.

Further reading

Gauhar UA, Gaffo AL, Alarcón GS (2007). Pulmonary manifestations of rheumatoid arthritis. *Semin Respir Crit Care Med*; **28** (4): 430–440.

Kim DS (2006). Interstitial lung disease in rheumatoid arthritis: recent advances. *Curr Opin Pulm Med*; **12** (5): 346–353.

Nannini C, Ryu JH, Matteson EL (2008). Lung disease in rheumatoid arthritis. *Curr Opin Rheumatol*; **20** (3): 340–346.

Ostor AJ, Crisp Aj, Somerville MF, Scott DG (2004). Fatal exacerbation of rheumatoid athritis assoicated fibrosing alveolitis in patients given infliximab. *BMJ*; **329**:1266.

British Thoracic Society Standards of Care Committee (2005). BTS recommendations for assessing risk and for managing *Mycobacterium tuberculosis* infection and disease in patients due to anti-TNF-α treatment. *Thorax*; **60**: 800–5.

Case 42

A 47-year-old man presented with progressive increasing breathlessness over 2 years, with an exercise tolerance of 100 metres, in association with a cough occasionally productive of mucopurulent sputum. His GP had tried increasing doses of budesonide and formoterol, several courses of antibiotics and short steroid courses with no benefit. He had stopped smoking 20 years previously. On examination he had a BMI of 46.4, no finger clubbing or cyanosis. Resting oxygen saturation on air was 94%. Respiratory examination revealed fine left basal crackles, and otherwise examination was normal.

Investigations

- Hb 15.5g/dL, WCC 8.01×10^9/L (eosinophils 0.4×10^9/L), platelets 267×10^9/L, ESR 8mm/h
- U&E, LFTs normal, ACE 57U/L (18–55), rheumatoid factor and ANA negative
- Pulmonary function (Table 42.1).

Table 42.1 Pulmonary function tests

	Measured	(% Predicted)
FEV_1(L)	1.3	40
FVC(L)	1.5	38

Patient unable to manage static lung volumes or gas transfer measurement

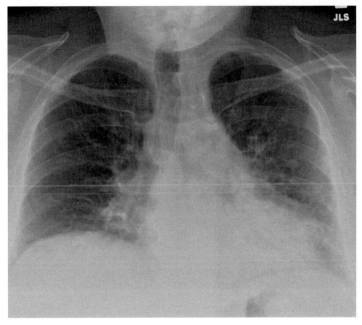

Fig. 42.1 CXR.

Questions

42a) Interpret the CXR (Fig. 42.1).

42b) What is the next investigation?

Answers

42a) **Interpret the CXR (Fig. 42.1).**

The CXR shows reduced lung volumes. There are reticular opacities in both lower zones, more marked on the left. There is loss of definition of the left and right heart borders and the left hemi-diaphragm. The heart size is borderline but the lack of septal lines or pleural effusions makes heart failure unlikely. Overall the appearances are suggestive of an interstitial process but no firm diagnosis can be made at this point.

42b) **What is the next investigation?**

The next investigation of choice is a high-resolution CT thorax (Fig. 42.2).

Questions

42c) Interpret the HRCT images (Fig. 42.2).

42d) What is the differential diagnosis?

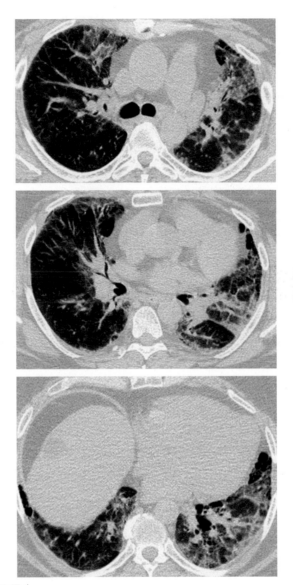

Fig. 42.2 HRCT thorax.

Answers

42c) **Interpret the HRCT images (Fig. 42.2).**

The predominant feature on the CT (Fig. 42.3) is bilateral multifocal ground glass opacity throughout the lungs. In addition, there is superimposed interlobar septal thickening, and areas of reticulation. There is no convincing traction bronchial dilatation (or traction bronchiectasis). There is pericardial fat, which explains the borderline cardiothoracic ratio on the CXR.

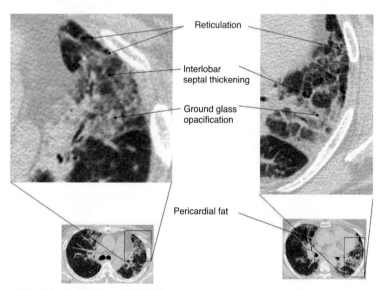

Fig. 42.3 Enlarged portions of HRCT.

The appearances are in keeping with interstitial lung disease, with reticulation and volume loss on the left suggesting an element of fibrosis. The lack of honeycombing and traction bronchial dilatation would go against a usual interstitial pneumonia (UIP) pattern. Mediastinal settings (not shown) demonstrated a 1.5cm lymph node just lateral to the pulmonary trunk in the mediastinum and further lymphadenopathy in both hila.

42d) **What is the differential diagnosis?**

The differential diagnosis would include an atypical appearance of UIP (with idiopathic pulmonary fibrosis (IPF) as the clinical diagnosis), non-specific interstitial pneumonia (NSIP), drug reactions, sub-acute on chronic hypersensitivity pneumonitis and (far less likely) sarcoidosis.

Questions

42e) Which of the following would be the optimum management strategy?

A. Treatment with high dose steroids (40mg prednisolone/day) for 4–6 weeks followed by tapering, according to response to lower maintenance dose

B. Transbronchial biopsy (TBB) + lavage followed by high dose steroids as above if infection excluded

C. TBLB followed by surgical lung biopsy if non-diagnostic

D. Surgical lung biopsy

Answer

42e) **Which of the following would be the optimum management strategy?**

    A. **Treatment with high dose steroids (40mg prednisolone/day) for 4–6 weeks followed by tapering, according to response to lower maintenance dose**

    B. **Transbronchial biopsy (TBB) + lavage followed by high dose steroids as above if infection excluded**

    C. **TBLB followed by surgical lung biopsy if non-diagnostic**

    D. **Surgical lung biopsy**

There is no right answer to this question. Purists would say C or D, and pragmatists A. However, most would argue that the management strategy at this point should be to establish an accurate diagnosis. The clinical diagnosis of IPF can only confidently be made in the context of characteristic clinical, physiological and radiological features (Wells *et al.* 2008). The absence of marked honeycombing in particular goes against UIP as the likely underlying pathology, as does the absence of other radiological features to suggest established fibrosis, such as traction bronchial dilatation. In cases of doubt, such as this, biopsy confirmation is required. Initiating steroid treatment at this point would not be appropriate as this could make subsequent biopsy difficult to interpret.

Choice of biopsy route is best guided by the most likely diagnosis. Transbronchial lung biopsy (TBLB) has a high sensitivity for diagnosis of sarcoidosis and cryptogenic organising pneumonia, but a surgical lung biopsy is best to identify the other idiopathic interstitial pneumonias.

In this case TBLB was performed initially given the radiological suspicion (albeit perhaps not high) of sarcoidosis. Culture of BAL fluid was negative and cytology showed no predominant cellular population. Histology showed two fragments of alveolar tissue within which there was some interstitial fibrosis, type 2 pneumocyte hyperplasia and macrophages within the air spaces. Patchy mild interstitial infiltration was present, but no well-formed granulomas were seen. Overall the appearances were not specific, and therefore a surgical lung biopsy was performed. This showed much of the lung parenchyma to be essentially normal, apart from two foci of interstitial fibrosis with some smooth muscle hyperplasia and focal chronic inflammation. No granulomas nor birefringent material were seen, and only occasional eosinophils were present. The apparent temporal homogeneity in the fibrosis was felt to be consistent with NSIP.

Question

42f) What is the most appropriate management strategy?

A. High dose steroids for 4–6 weeks (40mg prednisolone/day) followed by tapering according to response to lower maintenance dose

B. High-dose steroids and tapering as above plus azathioprine

C. IV cyclophosphamide followed by maintenance prednisolone

D. IV cyclophosphamide followed by maintenance oral cyclophosphamide and low dose steroids

E. High dose steroids (0.5mg/kg/day) tapering to low-dose maintenance (0.125mg/kg/day) plus azathioprine and N-acetylcysteine (NAC).

Answer

42f) **What is the most appropriate management strategy?**

   A. **High dose steroids for 4–6 weeks (40mg prednisolone/day) followed by tapering according to response to lower maintenance dose**

   B. **High-dose steroids and tapering as above plus azathioprine**

   C. **IV cyclophosphamide followed by maintenance prednisolone**

   D. **IV cyclophosphamide followed by maintenance oral cyclophosphamide and low dose steroids**

   E. **High dose steroids (0.5mg/kg/day) tapering to low-dose maintenance (0.125mg/kg/day) plus azathioprine and N-acetylcysteine (NAC).**

There are no randomized controlled trials of treatment in patients with NSIP. In the absence of any evidence to make firm recommendations, recently published BTS guidelines suggest a pragmatic approach basing treatment on the clinicoradiological profile of disease (i.e. most closely resembling IPF, organizing pneumonia or, more rarely, hypersensitivity pneumonitis). In our patient, whose distribution of disease on CT is similar to that seen in IPF, the new guidelines would recommend option E for treatment, although many physicians would adopt strategy B. This is based on the IFEGENIA study (Demedts *et al.* 2005), which demonstrated attenuation in the fall of lung function in IPF patients treated with steroids/azathioprine/NAC, versus steroids and azathioprine alone. A trial of high-dose steroid as monotherapy is not recommended in the new BTS guidelines, nor is steroid and azathioprine without NAC. Small observational studies have examined other agents, such as cyclophosphamide and colchicine, but their use is not recommended. As with IPF, in appropriate cases with unresponsive, progressive disease, lung transplantation should be considered.

Question

42g) What are the principle ways NSIP differs from IPF in terms of pathology, radiological appearance and prognosis?

Answer

42g) **What are the principle ways NSIP differs from IPF in terms of pathology, radiological appearance and prognosis?**

- Pathology. NSIP is characterized by spatially and temporally homogeneous lung fibrosis or inflammation with further subgrouping according to predominance of cellularity or fibrosis. IPF on the other hand, with UIP as the underlying pathology, displays spatial and temporal *hetero*geneity (different areas of fibrotic lung at different stages of evolution from normal to severe fibrosis). Dense fibrosis and honeycombing are present in UIP and a further pathological hallmark is the finding of fibroblastic foci in UIP. Formal diagnosis of NSIP and IPF must not, however, be based solely on the pathology, but on an integrated clinic-radiological-pathological approach (Travis *et al.* 2008).

- Radiology. Given this homogeneity with NSIP, the predominant feature on HRCT is ground glass attenuation with a basal predominance and subpleural and/or peribronchovascular distribution. Signs of fibrosis (volume loss, reticulation, traction bronchiectasis) can be present but should not predominate. Although honeycombing was previously said to be rare (Lynch *et al.* 2005), a radiological review of 50 cases of biopsy proven NSIP found this in 15 (30%), and bilateral in 13 cases (Hartman *et al.* 2000). Traction bronchiectasis was found in 18/50 (36%) and in association with honeycombing in 9. More recently, in an ATS report (Travis *et al.* 2008), with perhaps a stricter multidisciplinary concensus on diagnosis, traction bronchiectasis was relatively common (50/61 patients with evaluable radiology, 82%) but honeycombing unusual (3/61, 5%). Even in experienced radiological hands, there can be differences of opinion. In a study examining inter-rater reliability of 11 thoracic radiologists in the diagnosis of 131 patients with diffuse parenchymal lung disease (Aziz *et al.* 2004), NSIP was a frequent source of variation and involved in 138 (55%) of discrepancies. Overall the co-efficient of agreement was higher in this study (kappa 0.50) for IPF than NSIP (kappa 0.38). This emphasizes the general importance of seeking biopsy supporting evidence in radiologically suspected NSIP.

- Prognosis. When patients with NSIP are separated from those with UIP, in series of patients presenting with 'cryptogenic fibrosing alveolitis', several studies have found patients with NSIP to have an improved prognosis in comparison to those with IPF/UIP, and there seems to be further improved survival in those with cellular NSIP compared to fibrotic NSIP. For example, in a UK series of 78 patients who had a prior clinical diagnosis of CFA and had lung biopsies (Nicholson *et al.* 2000), median survival was better in fibrotic NSIP ($n = 25$, 52 months) than UIP ($n = 37$, 27 months). Three had cellular NSIP and all were alive at follow up. In the recent ATS project report (Travis *et al.* 2008) overall 5-year survival (67 patients) was 82.3%, and 10-year survival 73.2%. Despite this, however, it may be that patients with fibrotic NSIP, and more significant functional impairment at presentation, do not necessarily do much better than those with IPF/UIP. A recent study found that although overall fibrotic NSIP had improved survival in comparison to IPF/UIP after 3 years follow-up and longer, there was no difference in 'early mortality' at 2 years and this seemed to be linked to significant functional impairment at presentation (Latsi *et al.* 2003). There was no difference in survival between NSIP and UIP in those with a DLCO of <35 % at presentation suggesting, in this sub-group, biopsy confirmation is less clinically relevant (and usually impossible anyway).

Further reading

Aziz ZA, Wells AU, Hansell DM, Bain GA, Copley SJ, Desai SR *et al.* (2004). HRCT diagnosis of diffuse parenchymal lung disease: inter-observer variation. *Thorax*; **59**: 506–511.

Demedts M, Behr J, Buhl R, Costabel U, Dekhuijzen R, Jansen HM *et al.* (2005). High-dose acetylcysteine in idiopathic pulmonary fibrosis. *NEJM*; **353**: 2229–2242.

Hartman TE, Swensen SJ, Hansell DM, Colby TV, Myers JL, Tazelaar HD *et al.* (2000). Nonspecific interstitial pneumonia: variable appearance at high-resolution chest. *Radiology*; **217**: 701–705.

Latsi PI, du Bois RM, Nicholson AG, Colby TV, Bisirtzoglou D, Nikolakopoulou A *et al.* (2003). Fibrotic idiopathic interstitial pneumonia: the prognostic value of longitudinal functional trends. *Am J Resp Crit Care Med*; **168**: 531–537.

Lynch DA, Travis WD, Müller NL, Galvin JR, Hansell DM, Grenier PA *et al.* (2005). Idiopathic interstitial pneumonias: CT features. *Radiology*; **236**: 10–21.

Nicholson AG, Colby TV, du Bois RM, Hansell DM, Wells AU *et al.* (2000). The prognostic significance of the histologic pattern of interstitial pneumonia inpatients presenting with the clinical entity of cryptogenic fibrosing alveolitis. *Am J Resp Crit Care Med*; **162**: 2213–2217.

Travis WD, Hunninghake G, King TE Jr, Lynch DA, Colby TV, Galvin JR *et al.* (2008). Idiopathic nonspecific interstitial pneumonia—report of an American Thoracic Society project. *Am J Resp Crit Care Med*; **177**: 1338–1347.

Wells AU, Hirani N (2008). Interstitial lung disease guideline. *Thorax*; **63** (Suppl 5): V1–58.

Case 43

An 89–year-old woman presented with increasing shortness of breath over a 4-week period. This was associated with an irritable dry cough and lethargy, but no chest pain or constitutional symptoms. She had an extensive background history including ischaemic heart disease, myocardial infarction 2 years previously, left ventricular failure, mild and well-controlled asthma, and treated hypertension. She also suffered with short-term memory loss, which had been worsening for the last 2 years, and had been diagnosed as vascular dementia.

Her normal exercise tolerance had been limited for several years by a combination of left ventricular failure and hip osteoarthritis, but this had significantly reduced from 100 metres to 30 metres in the last three weeks. She was on multiple cardiac medications, had never smoked, and had no known asbestos exposure.

On examination, she was apyrexial, tachypnoeic (28/min), afebrile and had an SaO$_2$ at rest of 96%. Her venous pressure was visible at the jaw and there was pitting oedema to the calf bilaterally. The left chest was dull to percussion with absent breath sounds and decreased expansion, associated with rightward tracheal shift.

Investigations

Blood tests:

- ◆ Hb: 14.3g/dL
- ◆ WCC: 8.6×10^9/L (neutrophilia)
- ◆ Platelets: 372×10^9/L
- ◆ Urea and electrolytes normal
- ◆ CRP = 2mg/L
- ◆ Clotting screen normal.

Pleural aspirate:

- ◆ Blood stained, serous, no odour
- ◆ Protein = 48g/dL
- ◆ Glucose = 6.5mmol/L
- ◆ LDH = 478IU/L (serum normal 150–220)
- ◆ Cytology—no malignant cells, 40% lymphocytes
- ◆ Microbiology—no bacteria, no mycobacteria on ZN stains
- ◆ See also Fig. 43.1.

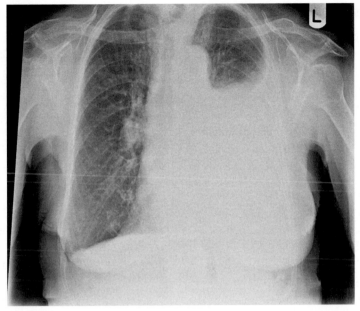

Fig. 43.1 CXR.

Questions

43a) What are the three most likely causes of the effusion?

43b) How would you investigate this patient further?

43c) How would you manage this patient?

Answers

43a) **What are the three most likely causes of the effusion?**

Given this lady's history of ischaemic heart disease, left ventricular failure must be considered as a possible diagnosis. The fluid is a clearcut exudate on the basis of the protein and LDH levels (>50% serum normal), which makes heart failure less likely as a cause, and the fluid is unilateral and bloodstained. However, up to 50% of heart failure effusions are unilateral (although only 33% are usually on the left side) and patients on diuretic therapy may have effusions which are classified as exudates on Light's criteria (see case 61).

However, given the size of the effusion (more than two-thirds of the hemithorax), and the age of the patient, malignant pleural effusion is the most likely diagnosis in this case. Up to 40% of malignant effusions will be cytology negative after a single pleural aspiration.

Pleural infection is a possibility, but it would be unusual to develop such a large infected effusion in the absence of other symptoms and normal inflammatory markers. Pericardial disease is a possibility, but likely to be associated with other signs and symptoms.

TB effusions may sometimes be this large; however, the pleural fluid biochemistry is against this (one would expect a low normal or low glucose level), and lack of lymphocyte predominant fluid is also non-supportive.

Effusion from pulmonary emboli should also be considered in an unexplained exudate (especially if blood stained), however again the large size is somewhat against this diagnosis.

43b) **How would you investigate this patient further?**

The investigation of a unilateral cytology negative pleural exudate is covered elsewhere (case 13). Invasive tests are likely to be required to obtain pleural tissue. In this case, considering the likely differential diagnosis:

- Heart failure—she is already on treatment for this and known to have a poorly functioning left ventricle
- Malignancy—in an elderly lady of poor performance status with short-term memory loss, establishing a diagnosis of malignancy is unlikely to alter management, and the benefits of chemotherapy are slim in most metastatic pleural malignancies. There may be an argument for establishing the diagnosis of malignancy for prognostic information.

- TB pleuritis is unlikely in this case given the pleural fluid characteristics—fluid was also sent for TB culture.
- Pulmonary embolus—a CTPA is a low risk procedure for this patient, and should be considered. However, management of warfarin therapy in this lady with short-term memory loss would require careful coordination.

One should consider carefully the risk/benefit of invasive tests to solely achieve a diagnosis.

43c) **How would you manage this patient?**

Given the above, a pragmatic approach to management is appropriate. Her heart failure treatment should be reviewed. Regardless of aetiology, she is currently symptomatic, and the effusion is likely to increase in size. Therapeutic drainage is likely to be required in the absence of a clear diagnosis. In a few cases of resistant and recurrent unilateral heart failure-effusions, pleurodesis can be a useful therapeutic strategy.

Progress

The options were discussed with the patient and her family, and the joint decision made not pursue a diagnosis. An elective therapeutic drainage procedure was planned, and given the size of the effusion, and the wish to minimize repeated interventions, chest drain insertion and drainage to dryness was pursued.

A 12F catheter was inserted in to the intercostal space in the mid-axillary line using Seldinger technique, and connected to an underwater seal bottle. Insertion was uncomplicated and pleural fluid drained freely.

Two hours later the patient began to complain of tightness in the chest and breathlessness, and then lost consciousness. Oxygen saturations were 97% on 4L inspired oxygen, blood pressure was 90/40mmHg and she was tachycardic (125bpm).

Questions

43d) What are the likely causes of her deterioration?

43e) How would you investigate/manage her?

Answers

43d) **What are the likely causes of her deterioration?**

Possibilities to consider in the case of patient with such symptoms after chest drainage are:

- Vasovagal episode—insertion of chest drains, and the associated pain caused by irritation of the parietal pleura, may lead to vasovagal reactions which are characterized by a transient drop in both blood pressure and heart rate, sometimes leading to brief loss of consciousness if the patient is upright.

- Re-expansion pulmonary oedema should be considered. This entity is generally believed to occur after moderate volumes (>1000ml or so) of fluid are removed from a long-standing effusion. Re-expansion pulmonary oedema is a clinical diagnosis made on the basis of typical symptoms (chest tightness, pain, and cough) in association with a drainage procedure. The mechanism is unknown, but is speculated to be related to fluid shift and loss of compression of the large veins in the thorax, or related to reperfusion damage in the expanding lung associated with vascular leak.

- Intrapleural bleed—chest drainage is associated with a low (around 1–3%) chance of intrapleural bleeding, usually due to laceration of an intercostal artery. Correct technique on insertion of the drain is the most important preventative measure (i.e. entry in the midaxillary line and just over the lower rib to avoid the neurovascular bundle which lies in the groove beneath each rib) in addition to ensuring there is no bleeding diathesis. The intercostal artery is NOT shielded by the rib groove until the angle of the rib—therefore posterior entry sites (around 4–5cm from the spine) should be avoided.

43e) **How would you investigate/manage her?**

Immediate management of this patient includes basic resuscitation (lie flat, obtain blood pressure, ensure intravenous access), which will not be covered in detail here. Vasovagal reactions will, in general, recover quickly and spontaneously on lying flat. Oxygen saturation should be measured, and the chest drain contents should be examined for evidence of blood or blood staining. In cases of doubt about blood stained effusion or frank haemothorax, a pleural fluid haematocrit is useful (and can be obtained on most blood gas analysers quickly). A pleural fluid haematocrit of >50% of the blood haematocrit is diagnostic of haemothorax. Thoracic ultrasound, if readily available, is a useful test to quickly diagnose intrapleural haemorrhage at the bedside. An urgent CT scan with contrast may be required in cases of doubt if the patient is clinically sufficiently stable.

Progress

Oxygen saturations were maintained, and after lying flat for a short period, the patient regained consciousness, although she still complained of chest pain and increasing shortness of breath. Bloodstained fluid was seen in the chest tube bottle. Pleural fluid haematocrit was 0.32 (blood = 0.38), confirming haemothorax. The 12F catheter was not draining further fluid and appeared clotted at the skin entry site. Her blood pressure remained low (80/30mmHg) and she was tachycardic (130bpm) despite fluid rescucitation.

An urgent thoracic ultrasound is shown in Fig. 43.2.

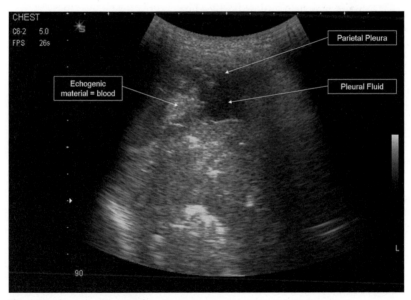

Fig. 43.2 Thoracic ultrasound.

Question

43f) How would you now manage this patient?

Answer

43f) **How would you now manage this patient?**

The diagnosis is a significant intrapleural bleed, likely secondary to iatrogenic intercostal artery laceration. Although care was taken during drain insertion to avoid the neurovascular bundle, the course of the intercostal artery in the elderly is variable (they may be more tortuous and lie in the middle of the intercostal space), and vessels are often ectatic.

Specific Management

An arterial intrapleural bleed is potentially life-threatening and unlikely to settle spontaneously—intercostal arteries may bleed briskly and tamponade of the bleeding point will not take place until massive blood loss has occurred. Plans for definitive intervention should be put in to place immediately:

- External pressure in the intercostal space of the approximate bleeding point may help to slow the bleeding.
- An urgent CT scan with contrast may be required, as above, if the diagnosis is in doubt.
- Definitive management is dependant on local facilities. Intercostal angiography and embolization of the bleeding point is possible where the facilities exist, otherwise thoracic surgery is required. In many cases, urgent thoracotomy is the only realistic treatment option.
- The small-bore drain is likely to block in the face of frank blood (as here). Insertion of a large-bore drain (at a different site) may be required, if the collecting haemothorax causes respiratory distress.
- Whether to remove the drain that has caused the bleed is a contentious issue—its presence may provide a degree of tamponade; however, it should be noted, as above, that a small-bore drain is unlikely to provide adequate drainage in the case of frank haemothorax.

Progress

Firm pressure was applied to the drain insertion site, and the patient was immediately transferred to the angiography suite. In transit, she experienced increasing respiratory distress and on arrival a large-bore chest drain (24F) was inserted. 1.6L of frank blood was drained immediately, with relief of symptoms. Angiography was commenced, during which she underwent a three-unit blood transfusion.

At angiography, the smaller chest drain was removed and the site of skin insertion marked with a small bead. The aorta was catheterized via the right femoral artery and the bleeding vessel located (see Fig. 43.3).

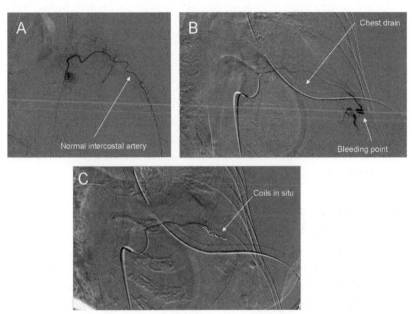

Fig. 43.3 Angiography and embolization of intercostal artery. Images courtesy of Dr P Boardman.

Angiography revealed a small pseudoaneurysm with active bleeding at the left intercostal artery over the drain insertion site (B). This was successfully embolized with 4 × 3mm Micro coils (C).

Further reading

Echevarria C, Twomey D, Dunning J, Chanda B (2008). Does re-expansion pulmonary oedema exist? *Interact Cardiovasc Thorac Surg*; **7**: 485–9.

Case 44

Six weeks previously a 75-year-old retired farmer had developed 'bronchitis' with a cough, fever and wheeze. Two courses of antibiotics (amoxicillin and doxycycline) provided little symptomatic benefit. Two weeks prior to his appointment, in late-January, he noticed his fingers intermittently becoming 'purple and cold', but with no associated white or red skin finger discolouration (Fig. 44.1). This only occurred when helping his son on their pig farm early in the morning, and improved a little as the day progressed. He had never smoked and was on no regular medication.

On examination, he had bibasal crackles on auscultation. Finger oximetry failed to register a peripheral arterial waveform or a valid oxygen saturation. Despite palpable symmetrical peripheral pulses, his distal phalanges were cyanosed (Fig. 44.1). His toes appeared normal. His CXR is shown in Fig. 44.2.

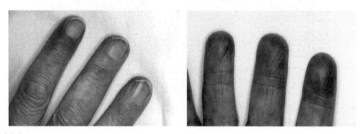

Fig. 44.1

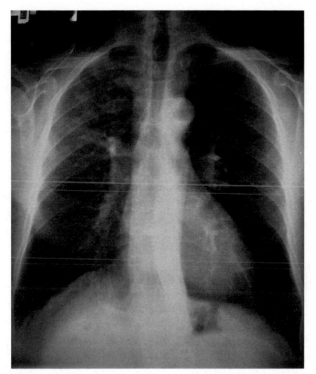

Fig. 44.2 CXR.

Questions

44a) What phenomenon is shown in Fig. 44.1?

44b) What does his CXR (Fig. 44.2) show?

Answers

44a) What phenomenon is shown in Fig. 44.1?

Fig. 44.1 demonstrates distal digital cyanosis. Raynaud's phenomenon is unlikely due to the absence of white and red skin discolouration, despite the fact that symptoms were precipitated by cold exposure. This kind of digital cyanosis is often called acrocyanosis ('acro'-meaning extremity or tip).

Acrocyanosis is related to reduced delivery of oxygenated blood to the extremities as a consequence of local arteriolar spasm or occlusion. The pathophysiology of acrocyanosis is unclear but is thought to relate to abnormally increased arteriolar tone, possibly as a consequence of elevated endothelin-1 levels, and increased whole blood viscosity. The persistent purple discolouration usually disappears on warming and there is little or no reactive hyperaemia. Acrocyanosis should be differentiated from:

- Peripheral cyanosis: associated with hypoxaemia, confirmed on arterial blood gas analysis, and central cyanosis causing mucosal discolouration
- Peripheral vascular disease: often determined from the patient's history, diminished distal pulses (e.g. pedal) and other signs of arterial insufficiency
- Raynaud's phenomenon: characterized by a triphasic colour change (white, blue and red) with associated pain and/or paraesthesia due to resultant sensory nerve ischaemia
- Erythromelalgia: a rare condition associated with erythema, warmth and burning pain of the extremities precipitated by heat exposure, alcohol, or exertion.

44b) What does his CXR (Fig. 44.2) show?

His CXR shows patchy right-upper lobe consolidation.

Investigations

- Hb 14.5g/dL, MCV 88.2fL, WCC 7.8×10^9/L (normal differential), platelets 387×10^9/L
- Coagulation studies, U&E, LFT all normal, CRP 27mg/L, ESR 14mm/h
- Fig. 44.3 shows the result of a diagnostic test performed on arrival.

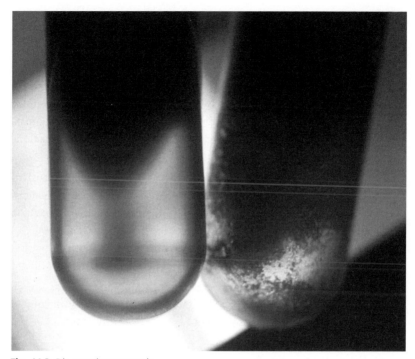

Fig. 44.3 Diagnostic test result.

Questions

44c) What is this test and what does it show?

44d) Suggest a unifying diagnosis.

44e) What further serological tests should be performed?

Answers

44c) **What is this test and what does it show?**

The 'bedside cold agglutinins' test can be performed to rapidly assess for cold agglutininaemia, i.e. blood in a tube containing citrate (or other anticoagulant) is placed in ice cold water or a freezer compartment for 5min and then assessed against a light for haemagglutination, comparing it to a warm control tube (Fig. 44.3). Haemagglutination is maximal between 0 and 5°C.

Red cell agglutination can be seen in the cold vial, which is consistent with a cold agglutininaemia and the patient's symptoms. Transient red cell agglutination precipitating acrocyanosis is particularly likely on peripheral regions where temperatures drop below 32°C. Gangrene as a consequence of transient cold haemagglutination is rare but a few cases have been reported in the literature.

NB: A falsely low haemoglobin level and high MCV may arise as a result of red cell clumping in the sample, and in this situation examination of a peripheral blood smear is prudent.

44d) **Suggest a unifying diagnosis.**

Mycoplasma pneumoniae pneumonia is the most likely diagnosis in this patient. *Mycoplasma* is responsible for approximately 20% of community acquired pneumonia and 5% of patients hospitalized with pneumonia. *Mycoplasma* infection is endemic, but punctuated by epidemics at 4–7-year intervals. It is about five times more common in smokers.

Cold agglutinins are detected in about 60% of cases and other extra-pulmonary complications develop in 15%, including neurological, renal, musculoskeletal, cardiovascular, gastrointestinal, skin and immunological manifestations. Other infective precipitants of cold agglutination include Epstein-Barr virus (infectious mononucleosis) and, less commonly, cytomegalovirus (CMV), *Legionella* spp., influenza, HIV, hepatitis and malaria.

44e) **What further serological tests should be performed?**

Serological tests that should be performed are:

1. *Mycoplasma pneumoniae* antibody titres. Peak levels are reached approximately 2 weeks after the onset of symptoms and decrease as symptoms resolve. Enzyme immunoassay (EIA) detection of acute and convalescent phase specific IgG and IgM antibodies are more sensitive for detecting acute infection than culture. A four-fold rise in titre is suggestive of acute infection. IgM antibodies against

Mycoplasma pneumoniae may not be produced during re-infection in patients over 40 years with pre-existing IgG antibodies.

2. A confirmatory cold agglutinin titre could be requested. Causes of cold agglutinin disorders may be classified as:

   ◆ Primary (idiopathic cold agglutinin disease) when the titre is very high (often >100,000–1,000,000 and associated with monoclonal auto-antibodies)

   ◆ Secondary:

     • Associated with monoclonal auto-antibodies, usually chronic, and related to B-cell lymphoproliferative conditions or non-haematological neoplasia

     • Associated with polyclonal auto-antibodies, usually acute and transient, often precipitated by infection, as in this case

     • Related to collagen vascular disease.

3. Complement levels (C3 and C4) are usually normal.

4. Direct Coomb's Test (DCT).

   Cold agglutininaemia arises as the result of specific immunoglobulin M (IgM) production (or less commonly IgA or IgG) to the 'I' antigen on erythrocyte membranes, which induces haemagglutination mainly at 4°C and not at 37°C. This commonly arises 1–2 weeks after the acute infection (as in this case) and is more common in childhood infection, decreasing with age. The titre gradually falls with treatment and becomes negative by 4 months. Cold agglutinin related haemolytic anaemia due to complement mediated red blood cell destruction may also arise. However, this is relatively uncommon given the inefficiency of the process in the absence of continued cold exposure, and is rarely clinically significant. The DCT reaction is usually negative with anti-IgG, but positive with anti-complement 3 in cold agglutinin disease.

5. Antinuclear antibodies, anti-DNA antibodies, anticardiolipin antibodies, cryoglobulins and rheumatoid factor.

6. Urinary *Legionella* antigen.

Investigations

- Elevated cold agglutinin titre 1:1280 at 4°C (upper limit of normal 1:40)
- DCT was negative for presence of bound IgG
- Antinuclear antibodies, anti-DNA antibodies, anticardiolipin antibodies, cryoglobulins and rheumatoid factor (<10IU/mL): all negative
- Normal C3 and C4
- *Legionella* urinary antigen negative.

Question

44f) What treatment should be initiated?

Answer

44f) What treatment should be initiated?

Empirical macrolide antibiotic therapy: macrolides remain the first-line therapy for atypical pneumonia, despite the recent emergence of resistant organisms in Japan. Doxycycline or fluoroquinolones are alternative agents.

The most effective treatment for cold agglutinin-induced acrocyanosis (and haemolysis) is avoidance of the cold. Calcium-channel blockers or α-receptor antagonists may be added and relieve symptoms in most cases.

Corticosteroids *may* have a role in reducing the severity of haemolytic anaemia due to cold haemagglutination, and cytotoxic drugs, such as cyclophosphamide, azathioprine and ciclosporine, have been successfully used, but are rarely required in acute infection-related disease.

Plasmapheresis can be used as an adjuvant, temporizing, treatment to remove the IgM antibody, if symptoms associated with acute infection related cold agglutinaemia are severe.

Progress

The patient was treated with clarithromycin and nifedipine, and advised to keep warm. His cough and acrocyanosis improved. At 6 weeks, finger oximetry showed good arterial pulsation giving a valid reading, and his CXR had returned to normal. A repeat cold agglutinin titre was 1:32 at 4°C.

List of cases by aetiology

Allergic/inflammatory	*1*
Anatomical	*21, 25*
Congenital	*7*
Degenerative	*14*
Genetic	*9, 11, 16*
Infectious disease	*4, 13, 20, 24, 31, 36, 44*
Inflammatory disease	*3, 5, 8, 10, 17, 18, 26, 30, 33, 35, 38, 39, 42*
Malignancy	*6, 19, 22*
Physiological syncope	*15*
Psychological	*12, 29*
Toxic/inflammatory	*23, 37, 41*
Trauma/inflammatory	*27*
Vascular	*2, 28, 32, 34, 40, 43*
Vascular/genetic	*34*

List of cases by diagnosis

1   Allergic bronchopulmonary aspergillosis
2   Hepatopulmonary syndrome
3   Diffuse cutaneous systemic sclerosis
4   Chronic *Haemophilus influenzae*, panbronchiolitis
5   Asthma
6   Malignant pleural disease presenting as ? TB
7   Pulmonary sequestration
8   Hypersensitivity pneumonitis
9   Lymphangioleiomyomatosis
10 Bronchiolitis obliterans/Chronic graft versus host disease
11 Cystic fibrosis
12 Hyperventilation syndrome
13 Oesophageal perforation and empyema secondary to TB lymph nodes
14 Shy-Drager syndrome
15 Cough syncope/chronic cough
16 Alpha-1 antitrypsin deficiency & COPD
17 Sarcoidosis and pulmonary hypertension
18 Chronic eosinophilic pneumonia
19 Hypothalamic lesion
20 Mycobacterium bovis infection
21 OSA
22 Mesothelioma
23 Nitrofurantoin pulmonary toxicity/UIP
24 Post polio syndrome
25 Primary spontaneous pneumothorax
26 Wegener's granulomatosis
27 Pseudochylothorax/Chylothorax
28 Pulmonary emboli
29 Exercise induced vocal cord dysfunction
30 Churg Strauss syndrome
31 Pulmonary TB
32 Chronic thromboembolic disease
33 Cryptogenic organizing pneumonia
34 Masssive haemoptysis in CF
35 Lymphoid interstitial pnuemonitis
36 Non-tuberculous mycobacterial infection
37 Severe COPD and surgical treatments
38 Upper airway obstruction secondary to Wegener's granulomatosis